The Parent Prep Book

Louisa Hirst

Illustrations by Sally Abel

2023

Where websites and organisations are referred to in this book it is crucial to regularly check these sources as research and evidence is always changing/evolving. Please also follow manufacturer's instructions when purchasing products.

This book is dedicated to all of the wonderful families I have supported in my career.

With thanks to my family, Hannah Croft IBCLC, Kathryn Stagg IBCLC, Karly Proverbs and Hannah Ewin.

In memory of Lucy Pedder who was kind enough to contribute to this book.

Contents

Introduction

Welcome to this book on all things babies and parenthood! If you are reading this you might be expecting a baby (or two or even more!), in which case "Congratulations" and I hope you're feeling well. Perhaps you are a Grandparent who is about to embark on a journey which sort of feels familiar but foreign all at the same time. Maybe you are a childcare professional who is about to work with a new family and you'd like to find out a little more about how best to support them in those early days and what to expect. Whoever you are I hope this book helps to prepare you for your impending arrival and ensures you feel more confident and prepared for this incredible and life-changing time.

Having studied at the world-renowned Norland College from 2004 – 2006 I didn't feel worried about the prospect of caring for my baby when I was pregnant. I had changed hundreds of nappies, supported breastfeeding dyads and prepared many a bottle of formula. I was far more concerned about getting the baby out than thinking about the aftermath. I have noticed that many families I support feel the same, not that they necessarily had ever changed a nappy before, but that they are so intent on the birth and delivering baby safely that the rest rather gets forgotten.

Now, don't get me wrong, I feel very strongly that setting out some birth preferences and ensuring you're as informed as possible for labour is important, but we must remember that this is only one piece of the jigsaw. You wouldn't get in a car and start driving on the roads without taking some lessons first. So why is parenting any different? Surely being as prepared as possible, understanding what is normal and having our expectations managed is not only helpful but somewhat reassuring when we might be at our most vulnerable? That is why I have written this book.

There is a multitude of books on the market around specific subjects, such as sleep and feeding, and antenatal classes where you can meet other expectant couples, but I want to take things right back to basics. I want us to think about why babies behave the way they do. What is it they're telling us? What is normal newborn behaviour? How have we got it so wrong in modern day society when it comes to baby's sleep? And once we know all of this we might then think twice before asking 'Is he a good baby?'.

You may not be concerned about what life with a baby looks like. On the other hand, you might be totally petrified and wondering where on earth to start. Or perhaps you just have a few unanswered questions such as 'What do I buy?', 'How do I maximise sleep?', 'Do babies just latch on and feed instantly?', 'How do I change a nappy?', 'How do I know what he wants when he cries?', 'Do I need a routine?' and so on.

During my time working as a Doula, I give information not advice and my job is to signpost to other professionals who specialise in specific fields, ensuring that my clients always receive the latest evidence-based information. That is why I have asked other professionals to contribute to this book and I am extremely grateful to them for their input.

I would also like to share some tips and tricks I've learnt during my career and whilst raising my own family. This is not going to be one of those books that tells you what to do minute by minute, hour by hour, but rather a gentle and simple guide through what to expect in those very early months, why these things might happen and what you can do to help yourself and your family.

Disclaimer

I recognise families come in all shapes and sizes with different roles and figures. I have tried to vary the terms I've used throughout this book, but if one of those doesn't relate to your situation then please do interchange to suit what works for you.

Chapter 1

Buying the Basics

Making decisions on what to buy for your baby can be an absolute minefield. From adverts on tv and Instagram to an internet search that brings up a million and one 'must haves'. It is so important to remember that babies are babies for a very short time and what we expect we will need very often turns out to be the polar opposite. So it is far better, in my opinion, to buy the basics first and add to things later when you know what you and your baby need. Let's face it these days things can be picked up or delivered in quick time.

It can be tempting to want to buy everything brand new but I would encourage you to think about saving the planet (and a few pennies) by keeping an eye out for your local 'nearly new' sale or online for good quality second hand toys/equipment/clothes. It feels so good as a seller to see items you've spent money on passed to a good home and as a buyer it's always great to grab a bargain! Granted, there will be some things you'd like from new but do keep this in mind for toys and clothes. Here is my list of things to consider. Please ensure that what you purchase complies with British Standards:

Travel

☐ Car seat- these are a legal requirement for children up until they reach 12 years of age or 135cm in height (150cm in Republic of Ireland), whichever comes first.

The seat needs to be brought brand new because you never truly know whether or not a second-hand one has previously been involved in a collision.

The first step is to find a car seat that fits your car and the best way to find out is to visit a retailer who specialises in car seat fittings. Please ensure you follow all manufacturer instructions. Some seats on the market allow for 360° rotation which means you can face the seat towards the car door making it easier to get baby in and out of the seat; much kinder on your back!

Babies and children are safest in their car seat in the rear of the car (with a second adult where possible). Ensure that if your baby is in a rear-facing child seat in the front passenger seat, the airbag is switched off. In the event of the airbag deploying the impact on the car seat would be severe. Equally, a front car seat should be pushed as far back as it will go, so that a child in a front facing child seat has less chance of head and chest injuries.

When placing children in a car seat ensure that there are no twists or slack in the straps and that the seatbelt buckle doesn't rest on the frame of the car seat as this increases the chances of it breaking and opening.

www.childcarseats.org.uk state that *'The top of the harness should be about 2cm below the shoulder of a child in a rear-facing child car seat, and about 2cm above the shoulder of a child in a forward-facing car seat. The harness buckle should not rest over the child's tummy.'*

Coats and bulky clothing must be removed before placing a child in their car seat so that the harness fits correctly (you should only be able to place one or two fingers between your child's chest and the harness). A child should never be left longer than two hours in a car seat, so if you're on a long trip take regular breaks. NB Premature or low birth weight babies are advised not to stay in a car seat any longer than 30 minutes and may need a special seat- ask your healthcare professional.

There are two sizing systems…

R44 weight-based seats, some seats of which cover multiple groups stated in this table:

Group	Child's weight	Age of child
0	Birth up to 10kg/22lb	Birth up to 6 to 9 months
0+	Birth up to 13kg/29lb	Birth up to 12 to 15 months
0+ & 1	Birth up to 18kg/40lb	Birth up to 4 years
1	9-18kg / 20-40lb	9 months to 4 years
1 & 2	9-25kg / 20-55lb	9 months to 6 years
2	15-25kg / 33-55lb	4 to 6 years
1, 2 & 3	9-36kg / 20-79lb	9 months to 6 years
2 & 3	15-36kg / 33-79lb	4 to 12 years

www.halfords.com, April 2022

R129 i-Size, these will take over from weight-based seats eventually. They are selected against your child's height. Babies in these seats face backwards for longer due to research showing they're a safer option for his weaker neck muscles (until the age of 15 months). There are three sizes, as follows:

0-85cm (approximately Group 0+ in weight-based system)	rear-facing baby carrier or baby seat using a harness
0-105cm (approximately Group 0/1/2)	rear-facing baby seat until your child is at least 76cm, then forward facing
100-135cm (UK) /150cm (ROI) (approximately Group 2/3)	forward-facing child seat

www.halfords.com, April 2022

I wholeheartedly recommend researching 'extended rearward facing child car seats'- these typically keep a child rear-facing until they're four years of age. When you read up on the benefits of keeping your child rear-facing for as long as possible you'll never look back. In some countries, it's the law!

Isofix involves the child's seat fitting into a base that is fixed to anchor points in the rear seats of the car, making for a more secure fit. The child's seat can then just be unclipped from the base (which remains in the car) when you leave the car and clipped back in before you travel. NB You will need to check if your car has rear seat anchor points before purchasing an Isofix car seat.

Impact shields are a new piece of equipment and are essentially an inflated airbag that fits around the front of the child in their forward-facing car seat and help to disperse the impact in a crash.

□ Sunshades for the car - something to consider if you don't have black-out windows. As lovely as the sunshine is it can be harmful to babies as their skin contains too little Melanin (the pigment that gives some sun protection). The sun can inevitably make babies very hot and also frustrated when it is shining directly into their eyes. You may find your car manufacturer offers these as an extra option so it is worth asking. Alternatively, you can buy ones that suction on or roller, but ensure they fit the window. In my experience the ones that slide onto the window are very noisy at high speed!

□ Mirror for car - this straps onto the headrest facing your baby's car seat and gives you a good view of them through your rear-view mirror without having to pull over every five minutes to check on them. Ensure it fits to the seat well or it will slide down as you drive meaning you have to stop to adjust it, making the whole exercise pointless! Some mirrors come with a night light so you can keep an eye on them in the dark. Please ensure the mirror is shatter resistant and has been crash tested.

□ Pram - for long walks and day-to-day you will want something that is reliable and solid. Most have lots of storage space underneath the seat for shopping and bags. For use in the first 6 months you will need a carrycot which attaches to the frame of the pram, allowing baby to lie flat in line with safe sleep guidelines and to encourage healthy spine and hip development. Once baby is sitting, he can move to a seat attachment. All-terrain wheels make it adaptable to all weathers and ground but beware of tyres as these often get punctures! It is best to go to a store and wheel some around to find which suits you best and which you find easiest to collapse and put up. Also, it is worth ensuring it fits in the car and around the house! Prams tend to allow baby to be parent facing or outward facing, but remember that parent facing is very beneficial to your baby's language development because you can chat to him as you're walking along. You can also buy adapters that allow the car seat to clip onto the frame of the pram, however, it is advised that babies do not spend long periods of time in their car seat. The Lullaby Trust states, *'There is no published evidence that states how long babies should stay in a car seat when travelling. However, infant healthcare professionals, safety experts and most car manufacturers recommend that babies should not be in a car seat for longer than 2 hours at a time and they should be taken out frequently.'*

□ Pushchair - having one can be useful as it is compact and lighter and is therefore useful for travel. Note that these will also have less storage space.

A note on Twin prams - same guidelines as above but note that the three-wheeled double prams tend to be easier to push than four wheeled. You can purchase side by side or tandem prams (one baby in front of the other). In my experience, side by side prams are easier to manoeuvre and as the babies grow they can interact with each other, however they are wide when navigating shops and buses. On the other hand, tandem prams are the same width as a standard pram but the babies can't see each other (perhaps helpful when you'd like them to sleep?!) and you do feel you're pushing around a minibus!!

□ 'Buggy buddy' - clips onto the pram/pushchair handlebars to hold shopping bags which is useful if storage space is limited- be careful not to overload though or the pram will tip!

☐ Rockit portable rocker - I have a number of clients who swear by this gadget! It attaches to the pushchair (or more lightweight prams) and stimulates gentle hand rocking. The only downside is it has a thirty-minute timer and then switches off.

☐ Rain covers - check these come with the pram/pushchair and fit properly as I have been caught out with this! Experience has taught me that covers with popper fastenings are more durable than Velcro. Also ensure there is always good air flow throughout and check your child regularly to avoid over-heating (you will need to be aware of what they are wearing when the rain cover is on and make sure they're not overdressed). Choose a cover that is made of BPA-free plastic as this is non-toxic.

☐ Foot muffs - helpful in the depths of winter but again be wary of what your child is wearing underneath to avoid overheating.

☐ Parasol - far safer than covering the pram with a muslin or blanket as these prevent good air circulation and cause overheating.

☐ Changing bag - many people tend to hang this across the handlebars of the pram/pushchair, so a waterproof bag is useful to help prevent the contents of the bag getting soaked on those rainy days. I have also found a rucksack is helpful as when you are wearing your baby you can pop it on your back, plus with older children you can be handsfree whilst running after your toddler!

☐ Travel cot - this is a lightweight, portable cot that fits into a bag designed for trips away. If your baby is young, you may use their Moses basket or decide to co-sleep but there are travel cots available that have a bassinet attachment if needs be, saving you from bending down into the cot. A travel cot is not essential to start with but useful as baby gets older if you're planning to stay away a lot. Ensure you find one that you find easy to collapse and put up... I have had many a battle with a travel cot and when you've just arrived on holiday this is the last thing you need! To save money you may be able to borrow one from a friend if you don't plan to go away much and some hotels/holiday cottages provide these upon request (you may need to take bedding with you though). Note: many travel cots come with a basic mattress which is woefully inadequate and I would consider purchasing a replacement mattress before use, ensuring of course that this fits the cot without any gaps. Please also check your bedding fits the mattress of the travel cot and that the weight limit is suitable for how long you plan to use it.

☐ Sling/Carrier - more on the importance of these later but there is an array of slings available on the market, from ring slings to wraps and soft structured carriers; this can be a bit overwhelming. Firstly, I suggest visiting your local NCT sling library and having a go with a few when your baby arrives to find out which feels the best for you. They will have volunteers who are very familiar with all the slings and how they work. The two main things to consider are a) is it easy to put on and take off and b) is it comfortable? The last thing you need when you're tired and potentially have a crying baby is to be fumbling around trying to put a sling on. Personally, I am in awe of people who use ring slings and wraps. Babies look so content in them and they appear to magically mimic the womb but I have found the majority of my clients get on better with something a little more structured that can be slipped on and they don't have to go through a process of tying together long pieces of material in a particular way. However, everyone is different and practise makes perfect so if you can make it work then absolutely go for it! Most manufacturers have online videos to show you how to correctly and safely use the sling, and don't forget to follow their guidelines on weight.

Sleep

□ Moses basket/Crib – The Baby Sleep Info Source (BASIS) state that the safest place for a baby to sleep is on a clear, flat sleep space close to their caregiver, day and night. For some people this will be a Moses basket or a crib. A crib is a small cot for your baby designed to be less overwhelming than the large open space of a standard sized cot. A Moses basket is smaller than a crib but is portable. If you choose to get one second-hand please ensure you get a copy of the instructions from the manufacturer and that it is undamaged and has come from a smoke-free home. The mattress must be brand new and it should be firm, flat, undamaged, have a waterproof protective cover and fit the cot so there are no gaps around the edges. Babies are designed to be with you 24/7 and often dislike being separate from you. I will discuss safe co-sleeping later but if this isn't for you another alternative is a bedside crib which attaches to your bed frame and allows baby to sleep next to you but in their own space. The bedside crib can be adjusted to different heights to match your bed frame. Note, The Lullaby Trust states that if you do choose to co-sleep you will still need a separate sleep space for your baby as babies should never be left alone in an adult bed without an adult in bed with them. There may also be occasions where, for example, you've drunk alcohol or taken medication which has made you drowsy, in which case the baby will need to sleep in a separate space. Please remember to follow manufacturer's instructions when using any of these products.

□ Cot – the NCT website suggests that there should be a gap of at least 50cm between the top of the mattress and the top of the cot sides to avoid baby toppling out, and that the cot bars should be vertical as if they're horizontal children can use them as a ladder to climb out. They state *'Also, the distance between the bars should be no more than 6.5cm apart so your baby can't get stuck between the bars of the cot. It is also recommended by some experts that a cot with bars on all four sides is better, as it allows air to circulate freely while your baby sleeps. If your cot has a solid head and footboard with shapes cut out, check that your baby's limbs cannot become caught in any of the spaces.'* You should always buy a brand-new mattress and if you're using a second-hand cot that you're going to revamp, ensure you use non-toxic paint and strip it of any stickers/decorative pieces that could present a choking hazard. Note, cots with drop down sides are not safe!

□ Mattress for Moses basket/crib/cot/pram carrycot - The Lullaby Trust recommends a firm (baby's head shouldn't sink in any further than a few millimetres), flat (not raised or cushioned) mattress that is brand new and complies with British Standards. It must fit the basket/cot properly with no gaps. Also, don't forget a waterproof cover.

☐ 2 fitted cotton sheets for Moses basket/crib (plus lots of muslins - these can be folded over and firmly tucked into the sides of the mattress under baby's head so that in the middle of the night, if baby is sick, you only need to replace the muslin rather than the whole sheet).

☐ 2 fitted cotton sheets for pram carrycot (again, plus muslins for spillages).

☐ 2 fitted cotton sheets for cot.

☐ 2 sleeping bags (choose tog rating depending on the season) OR 2 small cellular blankets and 2 small cotton top sheets for Moses basket/crib.

☐ 2 small cellular blankets and 2 small cotton top sheets for pram carrycot.

☐ 2 sleeping bags OR 2 large cellular blankets and 2 large cotton top sheets for cot.

☐ Red night-light with white/pink noise setting (more on this in the Fourth Trimester section).

☐ Baby monitor with thermometer and camera. Your baby will be sleeping in the same room as you, day and night, for at least the first six months but as he grows you will find a camera really useful when he goes into his own room so you can keep a close eye on him.

Feeding

☐ 12 Muslins (you can buy more once baby is born if needed).

☐ Syringes for harvesting colostrum (ask your midwife for these). They are 1ml syringes with a stopper on the end - again, more on this later.

☐ 3 bottles with Size 1 teats (bottles that self-sterilise in the microwave are handy) if planning to formula feed.

☐ Bottle and teat cleaning brush (I prefer the ones with a silicone head) if planning to formula feed.

☐ Formula powder (Stage 1 only in the first year. Don't worry about the brand as they're all very similar according to UNICEF) if planning to formula feed.

☐ Powder dispenser and Flask/Ready to use formula for outings if planning to formula feed.

☐ Steriliser/Steriliser bags (more on these later).

☐ Highchair - your baby can use a highchair once they are independently sitting up. It should comply with British safety standards, be sturdy with a wide base and come with a harness to keep baby safe. Choosing one with a removable tray can be handy as it's easier to clean and you can remove it and bring baby up to the table to eat with you. Some can turn into chairs and have adjustable heights for when your child is older, so will last longer. Highchairs with cushions made of a wipe-clean material are also handy. Double check highchair dimensions to suit your home and that you find it easy to fold away if needs be. Please be wary of the height of the foot ledge - your baby could use it to push themselves out of the chair. Also, highchairs that come right up to the table are a lovely idea but my concern is that they pose a risk for a baby to push the highchair away from the table with their feet and fall backwards.

☐ Breast pump (recommended to wait until baby arrives; more on this later).

☐ 3 Nursing bras (one on, one in the wash and one spare).

☐ Breastfeeding tops - you can buy tops specifically for breastfeeding OR just use something like a buttoned-up shirt or a jumper with a vest top underneath. This allows you to lift one material up and the other down creating space for your baby to access the breast whilst keeping the rest of you warm and less exposed.

☐ 3 Nighties with buttons/pyjamas with shirt tops.

☐ Nursing pads (you can get reusable ones).

☐ Multi-Mam compresses/Hydrogel dressings/Jelonet for moist wound healing.

☐ Expressed milk bags.

Bathing and Changing

☐ 2 Changing mats - 1 upstairs and 1 downstairs (or you could use travel changing mat downstairs).

☐ Kitchen towel for spillages.

☐ Changing station - don't forget safety straps to attach this to the wall so it doesn't topple onto baby. Ensure you keep nappy changing bags out of reach to avoid suffocation and follow manufacturer guidelines regarding weight limit. NEVER leave your baby alone on the changing table.

☐ Nappy bin - I have found the ones that twist and seal nappies inside, eliminating odours, are most popular with parents. Large enough so you don't have to constantly empty it either!

☐ Top and tail bowl- this is a bowl that gives you the ability to wash your baby without putting him in the bath, which is discouraged in the first few weeks of life. It comes with three compartments, one for water, one for cotton wool and one for discarded cotton wool. You can pick second hand ones up at a reasonable price from nearly-new sales.

☐ Cotton wool balls (you could use wipes made of water but be careful as I have found some on the market are very rough on baby's skin. The NHS recommends avoiding use of wipes until babies are 2-4 weeks old/6-8 weeks old if premature). When using water and cotton wool you may need to use a clean flannel or towel to dry baby's bottom before putting a clean nappy on.

☐ Nappy sacks.

☐ Nappies- 1 pack disposable Newborn Size One until you know size of baby.

Or

☐ Reusable nappies. These are nappies that you wash at home and although the initial set up may be costly they will save you money in the long run, plus they are kinder to the environment.

There are many to choose from so I have broken them down and given a brief explanation of each. You can find out more information at www.thenappygurus.com , www.thenappylady.co.uk.

All-in-ones: these are the closest to disposable nappies on the market at the moment. They have all the compartments built in – with an absorbent layer and a waterproof layer. They are easier to use as there is no chance of losing any parts or getting confused with how they work (a consideration if you have help with childcare!). The downside to these is that they take longer to dry.

Pocket: these are the most popular of the reusable nappies available. The outer waterproof later has a pocket for the absorbent layers to fit into. This is helpful as it allows you to build layers to suit absorbency level required. They dry quickly as the layers come apart for washing, however they require some sorting before use whilst you place the absorbent layers back inside.

All in twos: these have an outer waterproof layer which the absorbent layers snap onto with poppers. The outer waterproof layer doesn't need washing after each nappy change, unless soiled, so is useful for outings. It can just be wiped over, the soiled absorbent layers removed and new pads added. These nappies dry quickly as each layer dries separately.

Fitted: these are bulkier, very absorbent reusable nappies ideal for night-time and heavy-wetters. Consequently, they are slow drying so you will need a few of these. They are whole nappies made of organic cotton or bamboo, with an outer waterproof layer.

Flat: these are made of squares of absorbent material, folded and covered in a waterproof layer. The need for folding may slow you down but they are quick drying.

Additional items for reusable nappies include:

Disposable liners: these can be inserted into the nappy on top of the absorbent layers and allow for easier disposal of faeces, particularly useful once solids are introduced. They are also helpful during aeroplane trips and in the event of stomach bugs.

Reusable wipes: again, these reduce cost and waste. They are made of small pieces of cloth made of bamboo or towelling. You could also purchase them in different colours and allocate certain colours for certain jobs i.e. blue for bottoms and green for hands and faces! The wipe can be stored either in a box of water, ready to use, or can be wet upon use.

Buckets and bags: you can either use a bucket lined with a mesh bag, or a zipped bag to store soiled nappies in until it's time for washing. These lock in smells and are the equivalent to a nappy bin! You can then open the washing machine, open the mesh/zipped bag and throw the whole thing in. Normally the movement of the washing machine should remove all the parts of the nappy and wash them, but if yours doesn't then you may have to half pull out the nappy inserts (absorbent layers) before wash.

Travel bag: this is a bit like a toiletry bag, and often comes with a side for clean nappies and a side for soiled, ready until you have access to the washing machine.

Considerations: Velcro can get worn easily and catches fluff (folding one side onto the other can help with this but is another thing to remember before washing). When washing reusable nappies, you are advised to wash them every 3-5 days and rinse on a cold wash first (no spin), then a full hot cycle followed by a final rinse. Be aware that fabric softener and nappy creams can affect the absorbency of the nappy. Using a disposable liner in the nappy will protect any cream reaching the absorbent layer underneath. Sunshine is an amazing bleach for stained nappies so get those nappies out on the line! Squeezing lemon juice on them before they go on the line has also been known to help.

Always remember to follow the manufacturers guidelines when using reusable nappies.

☐ Oil for massage - the NCT suggest either cold-pressed oil or vegetable oil that is high in polyunsaturated fats. It is always advisable to do a patch test with any oil before use for massage.

☐ 2 Hooded towels.

☐ Bath sponge.

☐ Baby bath - a small bath specifically for baby which does not require a full bath of water. Alternatively, you could just use your sink, bring baby in the bath with you or use a baby bath ramp which allows baby to go in the main bath alongside siblings.

☐ Sudocrem Antiseptic Healing Cream for mild nappy rash, Metanium for more severe nappy rash. Both can be used from birth.

☐ Nail scissors - I have also spoken to clients who recommend using an electric baby nail file. Best to do this when baby is feeding or sleeping - it is a two-person job! Hold the finger or toe, gently press the tip underneath the nail down so the nail is free and trim across the top in short little clips. After a bath can be quite good as the nail is softer.

☐ Soft hairbrush.

☐ Bath thermometer, floats in the water and ensures you have the correct temperature for baby (between 36-38c).

☐ Coconut oil - I've seen good results shifting Cradle Cap with this as well as gently dry brushing the area, but always do a patch test first. Cradle Cap causes crusty/scaley patches on the scalp and face and is usually harmless. It is unclear why it develops but it CAN be a sign of allergy so it is worth keeping a close eye and considering if your baby has other symptoms.

Clothing

Until you know the size of your baby it is best to keep newborn clothes to a minimum. Remember also that you are likely to be gifted clothes as this is a popular choice of present for a new baby!

☐ x6 Newborn size babygros.

☐ x6 0-3 month size babygros.

> Lou's Top Tip: Babygros with zips rather than poppers are so handy, especially during those disturbed nights.

☐ x6 Vests (Newborn and 0-3 months, long or short length depending on weather).

☐ x2 Hats (Weather dependent and only for use outdoors, remove when feeding).

☐ x2 Cardigans or jumpers.

☐ Snowsuit (weather dependent).

☐ x2 Pairs scratch mittens (don't use when breastfeeding! More on this later).

☐ x2 Pairs bootees or socks.

☐ Bibs - maturation of the salivary glands can cause early dribbling so bibs can come in useful from a young age. I'd recommend large ones with poppers and a plastic backing, rather than velcro.

Other

☐ Baby bouncer - comfort and safety will be your number one priority here. I advise finding one that has different recline levels to suit your baby depending on their age (remember not to let them sleep in the chair though). Some babies like a bit of motion, others don't, so perhaps start with a second-hand chair to find out your baby's preference. It is also worth noting how easy it is to remove the cover for washing- some can be a nightmare. Please ensure you follow the manufacturers guidelines regarding weight limit.

☐ Toys - I suggest buying the following or asking for these as gifts as they'll all come in useful in the coming months: colourful books with flaps and mirrors
rattle and maraca
teething toys

a nursery rhyme cd
sensory mat or playgym
sensory toys e.g. feathers, light up ball, foil blanket, bubbles.

☐ Thermometer - the NHS recommend using an under-arm thermometer for children under the age of 5. These are good for travel but can be tricky to use as they involve the baby keeping their arm down for a couple of minutes whilst the thermometer works, something wriggly babies aren't often very happy about! Infrared thermometers seemed to come into their own during the Coronavirus pandemic. These are contactless and take a reading by being pointed at the forehead of the child which can be particularly helpful when they're asleep and you don't want to disturb them. Care must be taken to remove hair and perspiration before taking a reading. Ear thermometers need to be inserted correctly into the ear canal, and this can be tricky when babies have such small ears, but they can work well with older children. Marnie Doleman, a First Aid Trainer with the charity Freddie's Wish, suggested it can be sensible to discover your child's baseline temperature when they are well so you know what is normal for them, and to take an average when recording a temperature to ensure you get a fair result, as the temperature of ears can differ (particularly if a child has been asleep on one side).

☐ Non bio washing detergent- babies have very sensitive and delicate skin so avoid biological detergents as these can cause irritation.

☐ Family first aid kit- you won't necessarily need this immediately but it is definitely worth considering in the long-run, particularly for when you're out and about. You can buy them online or in the pharmacy. Remember to pop in some sachets of Calpol/Ibuprofen, teething medication, breast pads, an under-arm thermometer, sanitising water and a small pot of Sudocrem.

☐ Wall brackets - these help secure furniture to the wall to prevent accidents caused by tipping/climbing.

☐ Thermal mug - ensures your hot drink actually remains drinkable so you can enjoy it for longer even when you're rushing about.

☐ First aid course - I would highly recommend booking onto a first aid course antenatally so you are fully prepared for any emergencies that may arise. Always better to be safe than sorry.

Lou's Top Tip: Are you a friend or relative wondering what to purchase for a new baby... Why not spoil parents instead? Some herbal tea, some dishes for the freezer, a postnatal massage or a voucher for a Doula!

Chapter 2

The Fourth Trimester (or Fifth, or Sixth...)

So, you've carried your baby for nine months and you are told they must be ready for the big wide world by the time they reach 40 weeks. But is this really the case? Have we considered how we as human mammals differ from others?

The 'Fourth Trimester' was coined by Dr Harvey Karp in 2002 and is the term given to the first three months your baby is earth-side as he adjusts to his new world. For many parents the nine months of pregnancy can be a testing and worrying time and it can be incomprehensible to think that a baby is actually born sooner than they are ready. Your newborn will be doing the rest of his growing and developing outside the womb with you, rather than inside. And by recreating the womb world we are being respectful and supportive towards this transition.

It is also worth noting that a human baby's brain is only 30% developed compared to that of an adult, whereas other mammals' brains are 50% developed at birth. The human brain takes the most work to complete and requires the most input after birth.

When we compare different types of mammals it becomes clear just how different each of their characteristics are and it can be really helpful to remind ourselves of how we fit into this natural order.

Type of mammal	Characteristics
Follow mammal (e.g. horses and giraffes)	Well developed gross motor skills at birth. Eat solid food straight away. Can keep up with their mother. Milk is slightly higher in fat and protein than carry mammals as they don't feed quite as much
Nest mammal (e.g. cats and dogs)	Babies are left for chunks of time so milk is higher in fat and protein.
Carry mammal (e.g. apes, marsupials and humans)	Most immature of all the mammals and are totally dependent on their caregiver to provide safety, warmth and food. Milk has lower levels of fat and protein because babies feed very frequently
Cache mammal (e.g. rabbits and deer)	Mature at birth. Babies are left to fend for themselves so milk is very high in fat and protein

Now you may wonder why we as humans can't just hold on to our babies a little bit longer so that they come out more readily able to cope in the big wide world? Wouldn't this be so much kinder? Except the human body isn't built for that; whereas many mammals are stooped forwards, walking on two arms and two legs (or four legs), we walk upright on two legs and therefore have a smaller pelvis. This means that we can't gestate a baby long enough for their brain to develop fully.

It's also fascinating to note that babies are born with all the neurons they'll ever need. However, these aren't connected yet. The only way they connect is when a baby is fed, cared for and responded to and without the presence of Cortisol (the body's primary stress hormone). It is very important that as parents and carers we are sensitive to our baby's needs and responsive to their signals because this builds up trust, gives reassurance and aids bonding. Many people don't realise that this responsive behaviour also aids brain development and learning!

This is why we shouldn't only call it the fourth trimester; babies don't just suddenly stop needing us after this time is up. The love, responsiveness, security, empathy and stimulation babies need goes well beyond this time.

So how can we parent responsively and mimic the womb world? Well, if we think about what life was like in the womb it can help us:

- It was a dark red environment.
- Your baby could hear the whooshing sound of the blood rushing through the umbilical cord/your heartbeat/the gurgling of your digestive system/your muffled voice.
- He was weightless and constantly held.
- Your baby was naked.
- He received constant nutrition.
- Your baby experienced motion.
- His only smell was that of the amniotic fluid.
- Your baby received his sleepy (Melatonin) and awake (Cortisol) hormones from you via the umbilical cord.

So how can we replicate this on the outside?

- Red lighting for sleep/unsettled periods: not only does this mimic the womb world, The Sleep Foundation states that *'Red light exposure does not suppress melatonin production, so it could help to use red light bulbs for evening reading lamps and nightlights.'*.

- Play white noise/heartbeat sound during sleep times or if baby is unsettled (ensure this isn't playing too loudly or you'll damage baby's ears).
- Carrying: holding your baby or carrying him in a sling to 'wear' your baby helps you to meet his need for closeness and movement and also keeps his temperature, breathing and heartrate regulated.
- Skin to skin: www.unicef.org.uk states *'There is a growing body of evidence that skin-to-skin contact after the birth helps babies and their mothers. This practice:*

  - *calms and relaxes both mother and baby.*
  - *regulates the baby's heart rate and breathing, helping them to better adapt to life outside the womb.*
  - *stimulates digestion and an interest in feeding.*
  - *regulates temperature.*
  - *enables colonisation of the baby's skin with the mother's friendly bacteria, thus providing protection against infection.*
  - *stimulates the release of hormones to support breastfeeding and mothering'.*

- Swaddling: wrapping your baby safely in a blanket can help them feel secure. However, as discussed later there are risks involved with this relating to Sudden Infant Death Syndrome. It is up to each family to weigh up the risks, but please always check out Baby Sleep Info Source www.basisonline.org.uk for the latest research and follow the Lullaby Trust www.lullabytrust.org.uk guidelines which include:

'Never put a swaddled baby to sleep on their front or side.

Never swaddle when bed-sharing.

Stop swaddling (with arms wrapped inside the material) when a baby shows signs of rolling as they could roll onto their tummy and won't be able to roll back.

Use materials such as a thin muslin or thin cotton sheet. **DO NOT USE** *blankets or place any additional bedding over a swaddled baby, this could cause them to overheat.*

Ensure baby is not overdressed under the swaddle, has their head uncovered and does not have an infection or fever.

Check baby's temperature to ensure they do not get too hot – check the back of their neck. If baby's skin is hot or sweaty, remove one or more layers of bedclothes.

Baby should be swaddled securely to reduce the risk of face-covering by loose material.

Swaddles should not be applied very tightly around the hips as this is strongly associated with developmental dysplasia of the hip. However, the swaddle should also be secure enough not to come apart, as loose soft bedding can increase the chance of SIDS if pulled over a baby's head, causing a baby to over-heat or obstruct their breathing.

There are various swaddle products on the market for example swaddle blankets, swaddle sacks and swaddle bags. We can't comment on their safety but parents/carers need to ensure the products meets necessary safety standards. They should be well fitted.

Parent/Carers should ensure they follow the product guidance. Some swaddle manufacturers recommend their product is used when a baby is a certain weight, rather than age so it is best to check on the swaddle product they choose to use.

We do not advise on a specific tog rating for swaddle products, we advise parents/carers to use a lower tog rating/lightweight to reduce the chance of baby overheating.'.

- Bath your baby or bathe with him.
- Watch for baby's cues and act on these.
- Baby led feeding rather than a strict routine.
- Rocking/Swaying.
- Cuddling your baby whilst you bounce on your birthing ball.
- Limiting visitors- this can be a sensory overload for small babies with all the new smells and faces.
- Respecting the fact that babies have no idea of the difference between day and night in the first couple of months and that this will come in time.

All of the above will help produce OXYTOCIN, the love hormone, which helps stabilise breathing and heart rate, decreases crying and supports breastfeeding.

Chapter 3

What is my baby telling me?

Every baby is an individual and what is normal for one baby might be different from the next. Your parenting instincts are very powerful and will signal to you if something doesn't feel quite right. Don't worry if this takes time to establish, you are both getting to know each other. Babies are extremely clever and will give off other signals other than crying, such as facial expressions and body movements to express what they need.

A newborn's fundamental needs are:
- Love.
- Milk.
- Touch.
- Nurturing.
- Rocking.
- Ssshhing.
- Skin to skin.
- Cleanliness.
- Eye contact.
- Stimulation.
- Conversation.
- Sleep.
- Warmth.
- Body contact.
- Absence from pain and discomfort.

'These are the things that parents, usually instinctively, want to give but which some babycare gurus, family

members and society at large may seek to interrupt or prevent (even with the very best of intentions) because of theories about spoiling the baby or misunderstandings about why a baby cries.' Maddie McMahon.

As a general rule your baby's signals will look like this:

'I'm hungry'

Early cues are stirring, opening of the mouth, turning head to the side and searching for the breast/bottle.

Mid cues are putting hand to mouth, stretching and increased body movements. (Lactation Consultant Kelly Bonyata states *'After the newborn period, hand sucking is not as reliable an indicator of hunger. Starting at around 6-8 weeks, baby will begin to gain more control over his hands and will soon begin to explore his hands and everything else using his mouth.'*).

Late hunger cues are crying, agitated body movements and going red.

'I'm tired'

Staring into space.
Going quiet/still.
Yawning.
Turning their head away from stimulus.
Red eyes.
Slow blinks.
Rubbing his face on your shoulder when you hold him.

'I'm full'

Turning away from the nipple or teat.
Spitting the teat or nipple out.
Clamping mouth shut.
Baby comes off the breast/bottle of their own accord and
seems content.
Relaxed hands.

'I want to play!'

Wide, bright eyes.
Gurgling.
Smiling.
Eye contact as you talk to her.
Cooing.
Smooth leg and arm movements (as opposed to jerky).

'I've got wind!'

Back arching.
Irritability.
Crying.
Appearing to be in pain.
Drawing legs up to his tummy.
Clenched fists.

Lou's Top Tip: Give wonky winding a go... the stomach is a sort of a slanted J shape and wind can get stuck at the top. Place baby on your right-hand shoulder, with their chin resting on your shoulder blade and their tummy against your chest, and rub (don't pat) their back.

Colic

This is the name given to persistent crying for an unknown reason. There have been studies into the cause of colic but no one can decide what the reason is behind it. The most likely cause is an immature nervous system- think of the jump your baby takes from womb world to earthside. Babies have to deal with a huge change and often reach their limit by the evening, getting beside themselves. This is VERY hard for you.

So what's normal? Colic tends to start around 2 weeks, peaking at 8 weeks, and going by 12 weeks. You will find it tends to start in the evening and there is nothing you can do to stop the crying. Your baby may go red in the face, arch their back and get really cross whilst your breasts feel empty and you feel like you've run out of milk. You go through the usual checklist of nappy, temperature, hunger and cuddles but baby is having none of it. Then, all of a sudden, something clicks and they settle, feed and fall asleep.

Dr Ronald Barr, an American paediatrician, came up with the acronym PURPLE to help parents understand colic symptoms and what is normal. Typically, colic is determined by a baby who cries for more than three hours, for more than three days each week and for three weeks or more.

Peak of crying
Unexpected
Resists soothing
Pain like face
Long lasting
Evening

What is not normal is a baby who cries all day, who always appears uncomfortable, arches their back lots, isn't pooing (or if he does you find it's green/slimy), has a distended stomach, vomits lots or has a rash. Babies don't normally experience colic beyond 12 weeks.

It is always sensible to keep going through your checklist:
- Is he hungry?
- Has she got wind?
- Is her nappy too tight or has she soiled it?
- How is his temperature? Is he too hot or too cold?
- If bottle feeding, are you definitely practising paced bottle feeding?

- Is breastfeeding comfortable?
- Would you consider booking an appointment to see a Cranial Osteopath? Perhaps they have muscle tension in their face from delivery.
- Pop her in a sling and try some carrying.
- Massage her tummy and cycle her legs to relieve any trapped air.
- Have you checked there is no hair tied around her fingers or toes?

Teething

The NHS website states *'Some babies are born with their first teeth. Others start teething before they are 4 months old, and some after 12 months. But most babies start teething at around 6 months.'*

Symptoms may include:
- Red cheeks.
- Disturbed sleep.
- Excess dribbling.
- Gnawing on everything in sight!
- Sore, red gums.
- A mild fever (not over 38c).

The NHS website states that diarrhoea is not a symptom of teething and I learnt on my Gentle Sleep Educator course that the salivary glands mature between 3 and 6 months, causing excess dribbling which can easily be mistaken for teething.

As a Postnatal Doula I often get asked if I can recommend any products to help alleviate teething pain, and although I'd love to wave a magic wand or guarantee something will work, I can only share what other clients have said has helped in the past.

These include:
- Amber teething necklace/anklet (please ensure these are used safely and are 100% authentic) Check out @naturally.baby on Instagram.
- Sophie La Girafe teether.
- Brush baby camomile teething wipes.
- Matchstick monkey teething toy.
- Ashton and Parsons Infants' teething powders.
- Teetha teething granules.
- Anbesol liquid.

NB Please ensure you check with your GP or Pharmacist before administering any of the above and follow packet guidelines when administering.

You know your baby best and if you are at all concerned, please don't hesitate to contact a health professional.

Immunisations

Age	Vaccine
8 weeks X2 injections and drops in the mouth	(6-in-1) Diphtheria Hepatitis B Haemophilus Influenzae Type B Polio Tetanus Whooping cough + Rotavirus + MenB
12 weeks X2 injections and drops in the mouth	6-in-1 (2nd dose) + Pneumococcal + Rotavirus (2nd dose)
16 weeks X2 injections	6-in-1 (3rd dose) + MenB (2nd dose)

(Taken from the NHS website 2022)

Lou's Top Tips for taking your baby for their immunisations:

- Dress baby in something that allows easy access to their thighs.
- A Cochrane report published in October 2020 found that 'breastfeeding before and during vaccination injections helped to reduce pain in most babies up to the age of one year'.
- Premature babies will still need to be vaccinated at 8, 12 and 16 weeks from birth.
- Ask if the GP/Nurse recommends you administer paracetamol after the injection.
- Ask if there are any known side effects and what to look out for so you're fully aware and prepared.
- Don't forget your red book!
- Lots more information at www.gov.uk.

Skin

The white, waxy substance your baby is born with is called Vernix and this served as a protective barrier for your baby in the womb (to stop them shrivelling in the amniotic fluid, like we do it we've stayed in the bath too long!). It serves as a moisturiser for your newborn and a study from the National Library of Medicine found it even has antimicrobial properties, so it is best left alone/rubbed in, not washed off.

You may also notice your baby is born with, or develops, some milk spots called Milia. These are small white spots that develop over the face but are common in newborns and normally nothing of concern. It is unclear what causes these spots but contrary to the name it isn't due to milk. The spots are filled with Keratin, a natural protein found on the skin. As always, if you are at all concerned please seek the advice of a medical professional.

Umbilical cord care

After the baby's umbilical cord is cut at birth it is clamped. There are no nerves in the cord so this won't hurt your baby. After a few days the cord will change colour, turning blacker and hard/dry before falling off. It is best to leave the area alone whilst ensuring it remains clean and dry, and fold the nappy down to avoid irritation or urine/stools reaching the area. Keep an eye out for signs of infection such as redness or a foul smell. In this event medical attention must be sought.

Sticky eye

Due to their immature tear ducts many babies develop a blockage in the early weeks and you may notice a yellow discharge coming from the eye. So long as the whites of the eyes don't look red then a warm compress can be used to clear the area. Ensure you wipe from the inside of the eye out and only use one piece of cotton wool for each wipe to avoid re-introducing the discharge. Squirting breastmilk into the eye has also been known to combat any signs of infection due to its antimicrobial properties. If the problem persists or you are at all concerned, please seek the advice of a healthcare professional.

Fontanelle

The NHS website states *'On the top of your baby's head, near the front, is a diamond-shaped patch where the skull bones have not fused together yet. There is another, smaller, soft spot towards the back of their head. These are called fontanelles. It will probably be a year or more before the bones close over. Do not worry about the fontanelles as they are covered by a tough protective membrane.'* It is important to remember, however, that a sunken fontanelle can be a sign of dehydration so medical advice must be sought.

Centiles

Please seek help from an infant feeding specialist if you find the following:

Baby who was born below the 9th centile drops more than one centile space.

Baby who was born above the 91st centile drops more than three centile spaces.

A baby born between the 9th and 91st centiles drops more than two centile spaces.

Chapter 4

All About the Zzzzz

When we have a baby most of us know we aren't going to get the same amount of sleep as pre-pregnancy. And sleep seems to be the holy grail when it comes to babies. Everyone will be putting in their two pennies worth - websites and Instagram accounts claiming they have the magic answer or unqualified and unregulated sleep consultants charging huge amounts to help you get some shut eye.

However, I think it's really important to educate expectant parents antenatally so that they are better prepared for what is normal and have realistic expectations from the outset. Often, just knowing that what you're experiencing is normal can make a real difference to your coping strategy. Similarly, if you're reading this and going through a challenging time of sleep deprivation right now then I hope reading this will help to alleviate some anxiety for you.

I always like to start with a simple explanation of normal sleep physiology.

Firstly, I want you to imagine that within the brain, located at the back of the eyes is a solar panel. This solar panel controls lots of functions within the body, such as temperature regulation, urine/stool output and SLEEP, which all work in cycles.

As light hits the solar panel (our eyes!), messages are sent out around the body.

More light shining on the solar panel = the release of a hormone called Cortisol leading to a feeling of wakefulness.

Less light shining on the solar panel = the release of a hormone called Melatonin which causes a sensation of sleepiness.

So, you can see what a crucial role day and night (light and dark) has to play on the function of the brain (solar panel!) when it comes to sleep. Other factors affect the productivity of the solar panel too, such as temperature, noise and eating habits.

The hormone mentioned above, Melatonin, is passed from mother to baby in the womb, however once the umbilical cord is cut it is lost. Babies don't then produce their own Melatonin until around 12 weeks of age. Therefore, they aren't then able to tell the difference between night and day which explains why they can appear to have their days and nights all mixed up. Exposing baby to daylight and daytime noises will help support the development of baby's 'Circadian Rhythm'. The use of blackout blinds early on can disrupt this.

The hormone, Cortisol, inhibits the release of Melatonin and is produced in response to stress. So, it's useful when you need to run fast for a train, but not so helpful if you're trying to get to sleep. *Cortisol is a vital hormone, necessary for metabolism (Corbalan-Tutau et al., 2014), increasing blood sugar by counteracting the effect of insulin (Huybrechts et al., 2014). Cortisol also inhibits the immune system, reducing the inflammatory response (Wright et al., 2015), and acts as a diuretic.'*

At night sleep is driven by Melatonin, but during the day it is affected by another chemical in the brain called Adenosine. If you imagine sleep as a pressure gauge: at the start of the day the gauge is at 0 as we've been asleep for a longer stretch, and during the day the gauge starts to rise. Adenosine is produced as this happens making us feel sleepy, so we nap. During the nap the Adenosine drops, and the gauge goes down again. The cycle then starts over again. If, however, the gauge gets a blockage (perhaps due to baby experiencing feelings of pain or fear) then the sleep pressure is unable to work, and baby can't sleep.

The pressure gauge builds much more quickly in newborns than it does as we get older, hence why newborns nap so frequently. However, we mustn't be scared of this pressure building, we need to work with it. We can use this natural sleep aid together with a calming environment (which prevents that blockage) and our baby's unique sleepy cues to get some shut eye.

We need to be wary of sleep apps and charts, or those who assume any sleep issues are related soley to 'overtiredness'. Every baby is an individual. Some babies need less sleep than others. Some are perfectly happy after a cat-nap (these have been found to be restorative https://lyndseyhookway.com/2022/10/01/short-naps/). Some go from happy to exhausted in a very short space of time.

Tiredness cues can also be very similar to those of boredom, frustration or pain. Trust me that with time you will learn to read YOUR baby's signals.

Sleep Cycles

Once we are asleep the brain is working very hard. We actually all sleep in cycles. Simply put, these can be divided into two states:

REM (Rapid Eye Movement) – a light sleep known as 'active sleep' where baby dreams and is easily woken. Baby may exhibit grunts/brief cries/flickering eyes/jerky body movements. The brain develops and stores information during this sleep state.

Non- REM (Non-Rapid Eye Movement) – known as 'quiet sleep'. A deep sleep where the body is still and breathing is regular. During this sleep energy is restored, tissue grows and repairs and hormones for growth and development are released.

The length and order of these cycles changes with age as shown next.

Newborn

A newborn will begin his sleep cycle in REM, moving to NREM before returning to REM when they may then wake.

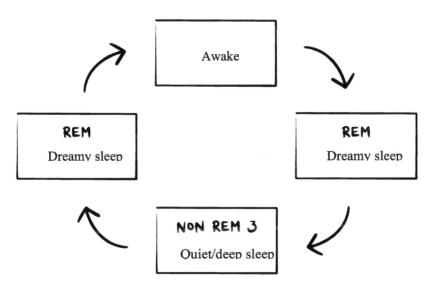

A baby's sleep cycle typically lasts 50 minutes, compared to 90 minutes long when a child is 3-4+ years old. So, you can see why babies wake frequently! These short sleep cycles and minimal deep sleep protect against Sudden Infant Death Syndrome.

Newborns may sleep for 18 hours or so a day, but only for a couple of hours at a time. They have tiny stomachs so will need to feed regularly, especially breastfed babies because breastmilk is digested quickly.

From 2 – 6 months

At this stage there is a shift in the stages of a baby's sleep cycle which can disrupt sleep. The cycle now looks like this:

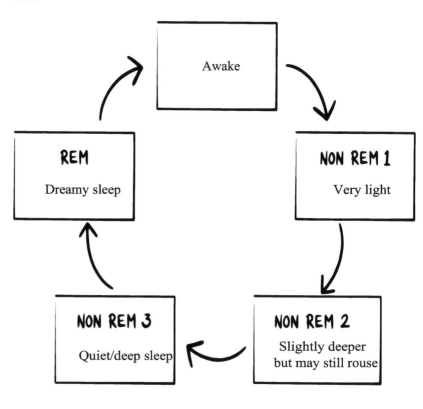

Not only do babies experience this change in sleep cycle architecture, they are also changing rapidly in their development, for example, learning to roll, trying to reach toys, becoming more interested in and aware of the world around them, and overall needing to sleep a little less than before. Your baby may want to practise these skills over and over both whilst trying to achieve them and once they've been mastered. People often talk of the dreaded 'four-month sleep regression' although there is actually a lot of PROGRESSION going on at this time (and it doesn't happen bang on four months!).

Lou's Top Tips for coping during regressions and broken nights are:

- Ensure there is nothing medically wrong with your baby that is causing them to be unsettled.
- Consider whether you wish to use the Wonder weeks app. This app acts like a calendar, showing you when your baby might be experiencing a so-called 'leap'. You put in your baby's due date into the app and it calculates when she might be going through some changes in development which can affect her mood causing 'clinginess, crankiness and crying.' Personally, my children didn't seem to follow the pattern on the app but I have heard others have found it useful.

- Respond to your baby when he cries.
- Follow your baby's individual sleepy cues and create a calm environment ready for sleep.
- Have a series of predictable steps used at sleepy time.
- Have a bedtime routine.
- Consider using white noise, familiar scent and red lighting at sleep time.
- Help her practise new skills, such as rolling and sitting up, as much as possible in the daytime.
- Find help from a friend, relative or Doula to allow you to rest as much as possible in the day.

6 months +

At this stage you will probably notice a pattern emerging, with most babies sleeping at fairly regular times during the day. However, they will still wake several times throughout the night and this is entirely normal in the first year (and beyond!).

Once your baby is sitting up solid foods will be introduced and many parents see this as the answer to sleepless nights as baby will be 'fuller', however, it is important to remember that the digestive system then has a huge adjustment to make that can sometimes cause discomfort and constipation or a higher stool output, not to mention the fact that your baby still gets the majority of her nutritional needs in the first year from milk.

It has been noted that some parents find that another common age for sleep regression is between 8 and 10 months but let's not forget this is when separation anxiety kicks in as your baby becomes aware that they are a separate being to you and that when you disappear you might not come back. During this stage games of peekaboo, always saying goodbye, offering lots of connection when you are around and sticking to a routine as closely as possible will help. It is also a common age for babies to begin crawling, teething and parents returning to work.

Pre School

It is not until the age of 3-4 years that children's sleep cycles mimic those of an adult.

Attachment

The NSPCC website discusses John Bowlby's theory of attachment; *'Attachment is a clinical term used to describe "a lasting psychological connectedness between human beings" (Bowlby, 1997)[1]. In particular, attachment theory highlights the importance of a child's emotional bond with their primary caregivers. Disruption to or loss of this bond can affect a child emotionally and psychologically into adulthood, and have an impact on their future relationships.'*

Newborns do not know they are a separate entity from their caregiver- when his/her comforting smell and body are gone, are they coming back? If we think about it, were babies put in the cave next door in stone age times?

With this in mind it is crucial that we meet our baby's needs. Babies cannot manipulate us and they cry to communicate something is wrong. You cannot spoil a baby by cuddling her, picking her up when she cries or paying her attention. Neither will you cause her to be clingy when she's older. It is in fact the complete opposite. By responding to her and meeting her needs you are showing her you're there for her, building up trust, confidence and a secure relationship. A child who feels nurtured will go on to build healthier relationships when she is older.

Self- Soothing

So, what about 'self-soothing?' Many out-of-date books tell parents that the key to a good night's sleep is to teach your baby to self soothe. Parents think they have caused bad habits and their baby isn't being 'good' if they're fed/rocked to sleep or if they're practising safe co-sleeping. However, for babies this is biologically normal. Self-settling is developmental, just like crawling or walking.

Self-soothing is a made-up term from the 1970s and is the ability to regulate our response to stress. If, as adults, we feel stressed or overwhelmed we are able to use the thinking part of our brain to think logically and problem solve to calm down. Perhaps we might call a friend, make a cup of tea or take some exercise. Babies, however, are unable to do this. This is because the upstairs 'thinking' part of the brain is not fully developed until the age of 25 years so babies, children and young adults find it difficult to regulate their emotions. Therefore, it is unrealistic to expect babies to self-soothe.

A baby who has had all his needs met and is in a calm state at the point of sleep will appear to self-soothe, but actually he just hasn't required support to calm himself from a state of stress. If, however, a baby is left to cry themselves to sleep not only do they learn that no one is coming to meet their needs but the stress hormone, Cortisol, rapidly builds up and studies have shown levels of this hormone remain high long after the baby has fallen asleep. This shows that they haven't self-regulated at all.

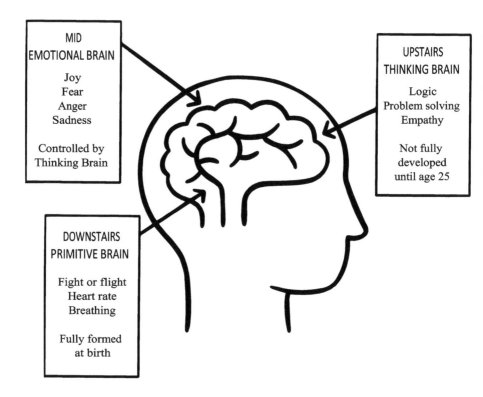

MID
EMOTIONAL BRAIN

Joy
Fear
Anger
Sadness

Controlled by
Thinking Brain

UPSTAIRS
THINKING BRAIN

Logic
Problem solving
Empathy

Not fully
developed
until age 25

DOWNSTAIRS
PRIMITIVE BRAIN

Fight or flight
Heart rate
Breathing

Fully formed
at birth

Sleep environment

As discussed above, your baby will experience an extensive range of changes in the brain during the first few months of entering the big wide world, not to mention a rapid progression in physical development which can cause disrupted sleep, but there are a number of things you can put in place to try to soothe her as much as possible by making subtle changes to her environment when she needs some shut eye. Ensuring the environment is safe should be your number one priority to help reduce the risk of Sudden Infant Death Syndrome.

Sudden Infant Death Syndrome, also known as SIDS, is the sudden and unexpected death of a baby that remains unexplained after post-mortem. The International Journal of Birth and Parent Education posted an article in May 2022 regarding a study carried out by researchers at The Children's Hospital at Westmead, Australia. It stated *'Researchers have identified Butyrylcholinesterase (BChE) as the first biochemical marker that could help detect babies more at risk of Sudden Infant Death Syndrome (SIDS) while they are alive. The study published by The Lancet's eBioMedicine analysed BChE activity in 722 Dried Blood Spots (DBS) taken at birth as part of the Newborn Screening Program, using only samples parents approved for use in de-identified research. BChE was measured in both SIDS and infants dying from other causes and each compared to 10 surviving infants with the same date of birth and gender....the study found BChE levels were significantly lower in babies who subsequently died of SIDS compared to living controls and other infant deaths. BChE plays a major role in the brain's arousal pathway and researchers believe its deficiency likely indicates an arousal deficit, which reduces an infant's ability to wake or respond to the external environment, causing vulnerability to SIDS.'* Dr Carmel Harrington, an Honorary Research Fellow at the hospital, who led the study, lost her own child to SIDS 29 years ago. Of the findings she said, *'Babies have a very powerful mechanism to let us know when they are not happy. Usually, if a baby is confronted by a life-threatening situation, such as difficulty breathing during sleep because they are on their tummies, they will arouse and cry out. What this research shows is that some babies don't have this same robust arousal response. This has long been thought to be the case, but up to now we didn't know what was causing the lack of arousal. Now that we know that BChE is involved we can begin to change the outcome for these babies and make SIDS a thing of the past.'* The next step in the study will be to add this test to the newborn screening when babies are born and to find treatment for any baby found to be deficient in the enzyme.

So, until such time, we need to take steps to make the environment as safe as possible for sleep. The Lullaby Trust recommends always putting your baby to sleep on a clear, flat space on their back (a baby's arousal response is higher on her back). It is recommended baby stays in the same room as you to sleep both day and night, for the first six months. If you choose a crib/cot ensure their feet are at the foot of the cot to prevent them wriggling down under the covers. Keep baby in a smoke free environment during pregnancy and after birth, breastfeed if you can and use a firm, flat, new and waterproof mattress. The charity advises not to sleep with your baby on a sofa or armchair, to sleep in a separate bed to your baby if an adult in the bed has smoked/drunk alcohol/taken drugs/is extremely tired/if baby was born prematurely or a low birth weight, not to use loose bedding or cover baby's face or head, not to let baby get too hot and to keep the cot or sleep space totally clear of pillows/toys/soft bedding/cot bumpers. Items such as sleep pods/nests aren't recommended as they can lead to overheating. Any cot, crib or Moses basket should be kept away from heaters/radiators, blind cords, wall decorations/pictures, other furniture that baby could clamber onto and direct sunlight. Hot water bottles and electric blankets must be avoided. If your baby is sleeping in their pram during the day inside, then the hood needs to be put down to allow for circulation.

The Durham Infancy and Sleep Centre state on their website *'...some research has suggested that swaddling might not always be safe: Babies that are swaddled may sleep more deeply. While this may at first appear to be a good thing it may in fact put them at higher risk of SIDS. The ability to arouse (begin to wake) from sleep is key to a baby's ability to cope with things in their environment that might otherwise put them at risk of SIDS.'* It is therefore up to parents to make an informed choice.

- Gentle white noise in the first 6 months, Alpha music thereafter. Alpha music is music recorded to a resting pulse rate, helping the brainwaves to relax. You can find specific white noise/alpha music CDs, or 8 hour playlists on apps such as You Tube and Spotify. Don't forget to ensure it plays continuously all night to support them as they transition through sleep cycles! The Hatch Rest doubles up as a sound machine and a night light that can be set on a timer.
- Temp of room- the ideal room temperature is between 16 and 20°c. You can buy baby monitors with a thermometer reading or buy a room thermometer separately. Keep an eye on your baby's temperature by feeling the back of their neck or chest. If they feel hot, sweaty or clammy then layers will need to be removed. Note that

younger baby's hands and feet might feel colder due to their immature circulatory system. During summer months keep curtains and windows shut during the day and place a fan in the corner of the room during sleepy time to keep air flowing (just ensure it's not pointing directly at the baby). A cooler room and layered clothing are recommended as you can then add or remove depending on the temperature, but a sleeping bag is another option as these come in different tog ratings. Always follow the manufacturer guidelines on which tog to use in which temperature, recommended weight of baby for the bag and how many layers to dress baby in underneath (blankets must not be used at the same time). The bag must fit securely around the neck so there is no risk of him wriggling down into it. Remember if you're using a blanket/sheet instead and it is folded in half it counts as two layers and these should be tucked in firmly to the mattress and below baby's shoulder level.

- Swaddling – please take a look at the safe swaddling guidelines in Chapter 2, plus the section on SIDS above. Here's my step-by-step guide on how to swaddle your baby if you choose to do so:

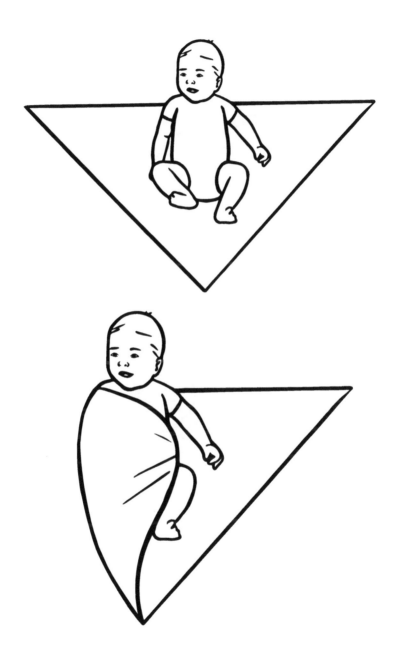

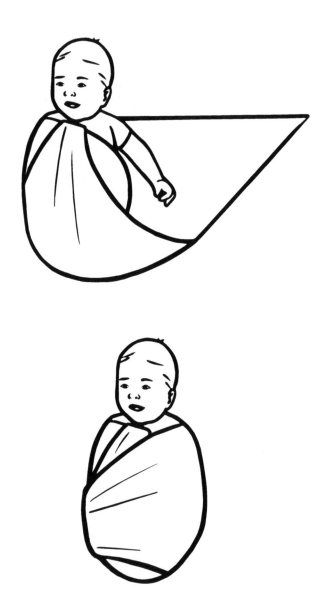

- Bedsharing - Sharing a bed with your baby is another option (NOT recommended for premature or low birth weight babies under 5.5 lbs). You can buy cots that attach onto the frame of your bed that allow easy access to your baby for feeding whilst allowing you to slide her back into her own space once she is asleep. This is known as co-sleeping. But if you'd rather have your baby in bed with you, known as bedsharing, there are a number of recommendations to follow to keep her safe. These include placing baby on their back to sleep and remaining with them at all times, not swaddling your baby and using a sleeping bag instead, not sharing a bed if an adult in the bed smokes/has taken drugs or alcohol/is taking medication that makes you drowsy, making sure the space where your baby is sleeping is clear of your pillows/duvets/pyjamas and remembering to tie your hair back if it's long. Adopting a natural 'cuddle curl' can keep your baby safe by preventing them from wriggling up or down the bed. This involves creating a c-shape around the top of your baby with the arm you're lying on and bringing your knees up underneath baby with your back to your partner. Ensure there are no pets or other children in the bed or any gaps baby could get stuck in. If your baby's head sinks down into the bed mattress more than a few millimetres then you will need a firmer one. Note if you are bottle feeding: https://www.basisonline.org.uk/hcp-bed-sharing-and-non-breastfeeders/

- A transitional object such as a bamboo comforter can be really helpful once your baby is over six months of age as it can provide a bridge between you and baby whilst transitioning into the cot and during sleep time. A few days before you give it to your baby tuck it into your bra or sleep with it overnight so it takes on your smell. For a baby under the age of six months you can sleep with a muslin and the following day fold it in half and tuck it tightly into the crib mattress under her head so she can smell you.
- The right lighting is key for sleep. As mentioned earlier, red light prevents the suppression of the release of Melatonin (sleepy hormone) so is less likely to cause wakefulness, unlike blue light. It can be really helpful to have red lighting during bath time too, after all lying in a bath staring at the ceiling right at a blue light bulb is not going to help anyone feel tired!
- Starting a bedtime routine from around the three-month mark, once the circadian rhythm kicks in, can be a really helpful tool in setting the scene for sleep and give some predictability to help give your child a sense of security. You will naturally begin to notice your baby falling asleep at a similar time each night so you can use this to create a sequence of consistent steps leading up to this moment. You'll need the room baby is sleeping in prepared with red lighting and white noise playing, and if baby is sleeping in a separate space to you either a muslin smelling of you tucked into the mattress, or their comforter at the ready if

they're over 6 months. Next, you'll give baby a bath, followed by a massage, pjs on and then milk/cuddles/rock/pat. You can incorporate a story into the routine as your child gets older too. At nap time you can follow a mini version of these steps.

- Creating CALM- this is done by ensuring the steps in the sequence are calming, e.g. no noisy, squeaky books or blue lighting!
- Get outside for lots of fresh air and daylight to support the development of the circadian rhythm, whilst also stimulating your baby's brain development.
- Remember that touch and baby massage aid sleep as they reduce Cortisol levels and raise Oxytocin so give this a go.
- If you need to transfer baby to a separate sleep space pop them in bottom first, gradually lowering them with a gentle rock/pat. When they are then lying flat keep your hands on their chest for a little while, so they know you're close.

Average sleep charts

When looking at these charts it is important to note that these are only an average, and many babies sleep patterns will differ. However, I have still added one here as I recognise that some parents find comfort in having something to refer to;

Age	Number of naps	Total length of naptime hours	Night-time sleep hours*	Total of night-time and naptime sleep
Newborn	-	-	-	16-18 hours (6 - 7 sleep periods)
3 months	3	5 – 6	10 – 11	15
6 months	2	3 – 4	10 – 11	14 – 15
9 months	2	2.5 – 4	11 – 12	14
12 months	1 – 2	2 – 3	11.5 – 12	13.5 – 14

*These averages don't signify unbroken stretches of sleep since night waking is normal.

© Elizabeth Pantley, The No-Cry Sleep Solution and The No-Cry Sleep Solution for Toddlers & Preschoolers (McGraw-Hill)

Chapter 5

Breast/Chest Feeding

As a Doula I pride myself in supporting parents no matter how they parent, and how they choose to feed their baby is no different. When I run antenatal classes I want clients to leave feeling fully informed and comfortable with their decision and that's my aim for the next two chapters. I would highly recommend seeking out your local International Certified Lactation Consultant (IBCLC), Breastfeeding Counsellor or Peer Supporter who can support you with any worries or concerns you have. These professionals can support you with both breast AND bottle feeding.

An IBCLC holds the gold standard qualification in breastfeeding and can help with all manner of issues including the more complex situations. They have to sit an exam and prior to this they must have had 1000 hours of clinical experience and at least 90 hours of advanced lactation education. An IBCLC is usually a healthcare professional or someone who has studied 14 health science subjects. They must demonstrate they are keeping up to date with the latest evidence-based practise, recertifying every five years, and adhere to professional standards.

A Breastfeeding Counsellor has usually trained through a charity and offers voluntary support for common breastfeeding problems. However, some choose to pay privately to train; just remember to check out their qualifications are legitimate before you meet them.

A Peer Supporter or Breastfeeding Buddy is usually someone who has breastfed their own baby and has had 16-36 hours of breastfeeding education. They will be there as your cheerleader, encouraging and supporting you with the basics of breastfeeding.

Breastfeeding provides health benefits to both you and your baby.

Baby

- It contains antibodies from illnesses that you have been exposed to.
- It lines the intestinal tract which prevents many foreign proteins passing through.
- It contains enzymes that support digestion and the absorption of nutrients.
- It kills harmful micro-organisms.
- It aids the expulsion of your baby's first poo (Meconium) which helps prevent Jaundice as your baby poos out Bilirubin.
- The World Health Organisation suggests breastfed children have a higher IQ and are less likely to be obese as adults.

<u>You</u>

- Helps protect against Ovarian/Breast Cancer and Heart Disease.
- Lowers the risk of Osteoporosis.
- Burns calories.
- Helps the uterus contract back to normal size.
- Kinder on the purse strings.

Due to this reduction in disease and illness there is less pressure on GPs and the NHS and breastfeeding is also better for the environment as there is no packaging, distribution or energy required in the manufacturing. It is ready made and ready to go!

Breastfeeding doesn't always come naturally to parents and it is something both you and your baby need to learn, but by equipping yourself with as much knowledge and information as possible antenatally, plus lining up the right support when your baby arrives, you are giving yourself the best chance of success.

You can start to prepare for breastfeeding by hand expressing your baby's first milk, called Colostrum, and harvesting this whilst you're pregnant from about 36 weeks (for multiple/high-risk pregnancies ask your healthcare professional first, not advised for anyone with a cervical stitch/incompetence or a history of threatened or actual premature labour). Hand expressing is a really useful skill to learn antenatally when hopefully you've got a little more time and having some colostrum ready and waiting when baby arrives can be super handy if your baby is very sleepy after birth as this gives them a boost of energy which will hopefully be what they need to come to the breast and feed. Your baby might also require supplementary feeds due to medication or congenital conditions, so to have a safety net there can be very reassuring.

To begin hand expressing firstly you need to wash your hands. You will need a 1ml syringe with a stopper in the end (ask your midwife for some) and a sterile spoon. Then you need to set the scene; a lovely Oxytocin filled environment where you feel relaxed is key, similar to that of conception! Oxytocin is the hormone responsible for the expulsion of milk so it's going to be your best friend over the next few months/years! You might like to close the curtains, light a candle, put some music on and sit with a scan photo and once you're relaxed you can begin to massage the breast. Gently stroke around the breast or make your hand into a fist and make rolling movements. Nipple stimulation might also do the trick. Then you're going to make a c shape with your thumb and index finger either side of the nipple and then work your way back from the nipple to just beyond the edge of the areola where you will find a knobbly part- this is different on each person so have a feel around until you find it.

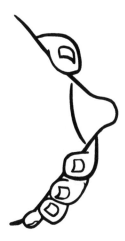

Next you're going to push your thumb and finger back towards the chest wall, squeeze them together and release.

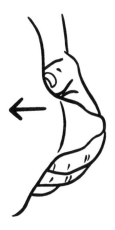

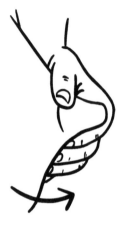

Repeat this and you will get a good rhythm going. Be careful not to draw the colostrum out and squeeze the nipple as this can damage the skin and make you sore. If you notice some beads of colostrum appearing, you can catch these onto a sterile spoon and draw these up into a syringe to pop in the freezer. You can add colostrum to the same syringe over a period of 24 hours, storing it in the fridge, before it then needs to go in the freezer. Or you can draw the colostrum directly from the breast into the syringe. Once you have spent a little bit of time massaging one area of the breast you can work your thumb and finger around the breast to another part, imagining the breast was a clock face. Push towards the chest wall, squeeze and release again.

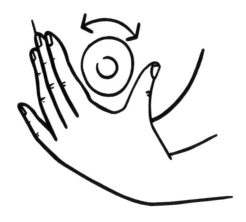

Once you have spent about five minutes on one breast move to the other side and repeat exactly the same process. Don't worry if you don't produce any colostrum during the first few times of trying, or indeed none at all before your baby arrives. This is normal and doesn't mean you won't produce milk for your baby. Start off by hand expressing once or twice a day from 36 weeks, working up to four to five times a day towards baby's due date. You can transport the syringes with you into hospital in a cool box for finger feeding when your baby arrives, just remember to put your name, date and hospital number on the syringe and ensure the midwives know it's yours and where it is kept. Defrost by running under warm water.

As soon as your baby is born, he will be put onto your chest skin to skin with a warm towel placed over the top. Newborn reflexes are behaviours that a baby is born with and are in response to a certain action. They allow a baby to find his way to the breast when placed on his mother's chest, latch and obtain milk. The baby just needs the right conditions and opportunities for this to happen. A healthy term baby is born with three main reflexes and these are: Rooting- baby turns head when feeling stimulus on his cheek, then moves towards the stimulus, finding the nipple. Sucking- if something is far enough into the baby's mouth they'll suckle. Swallowing- once enough milk is in the baby's mouth he swallows.

Having your baby skin to skin has many incredible benefits for you both:

- Reduces stress levels- release of endorphins and an anaesthetic effect.
- Initiates strong, instinctive behaviours and reflexes within baby to feed.
- Colonisation of baby's skin with friendly bacteria of nursing parent's skin.
- Energy used to grow and gain weight instead of maintaining temperature/crying. Baby feels warm, safe and content.
- Stimulates Oxytocin and Prolactin in the nursing person- leading to milk production, bonding, parenting instincts and confidence.
- Regulation of temperature, heartrate and breathing in the baby.

You may have heard of something called 'The Golden Hour'. This is an allocated period of time that if all is well with mother a baby after the birth, they are left undisturbed. However, if anyone tries to talk to you about this hour they need to be corrected. There should be no limit on the time a baby is 'allowed' to try and have their first feed. Time and respect should be given to allow uninterrupted and unhurried time on the mother's chest, allowing optimum conditions for the baby to elicit natural behaviours and reflexes to attach to the breast. This process is called imprinting and if any of these points are disturbed he will have to start back at the beginning, causing him to lose valuable skills and time. All checks of mother and baby can be done during skin to skin.

Given the right conditions, the nine instinctive behaviours a newborn will go through look like this:

Birth cry- baby doesn't necessarily cry but this is baby's first breath and inflation of their lungs

↓

Relaxation- the baby is skin to skin and can hear the mother's heartbeat

↓

Awakening- from about ten minutes after birth. Baby becomes alert, opens her eyes and Mum can look at her

↓

Activity- movement of the baby's arms and pushing across the nursing parent's chest with their feet- making their way to the breast

↓

Rest- This time should not be rushed. Baby may start moving and then rest again, repeatedly. Follow the baby

↓

Crawling- Making their way to the breast

↓

Familiarisation- Hands touching the breast and opening/closing their hands which stimulates Oxytocin and the baby's reflexes. Bobbing their head which will help erect nipple so it is easier for the baby to root for. The baby is using the sensations of the breast and nipple on their cheek to navigate where they are going. The baby may stick their tongue out/lick the breast

↓

Suckling- as soon as the nipple touches the palate the baby will suck and then when his mouth is full of milk he will swallow

↓

Sleeping

I find it fascinating that the Montgomery glands on the areola secrete a substance that smells just like the amniotic fluid in the womb, so it smells like home to your little one. Babies have special pressure points on the front of their bodies that help turn on the nine instinctive feeding behaviours. Having full contact with your body, lying back using gravity as your friend, triggers these behaviours. Medication and labour can negatively impact these inbuilt behaviours so ensure you have support from your birth partner/doula/midwife to help you get started, and if you are separated from your baby your priority will be to protect your milk supply by hand expressing at least 8-10 times in 24 hours. Remember midwife educator Carla Hartley's phrase during this undisturbed time; *'No hatting, patting or chatting...!'* Leave baby alone to do their thing! Unlimited and early access to the breast determines a mother's capacity for long term milk production.

Babies are born with very small stomachs and it is common for antenatal classes to show pictures of cherries, walnuts and ping pong balls to demonstrate the change in size of the stomach as baby grows. However, just like us, all newborns are individual and what a baby consumes is not linear and there is a wide range of normal. There are many factors that affect how much a baby takes such as type of delivery, the weight of the baby, how breastfeeding is going and if the nursing parent has breastfed before.

Additionally, the cherries and walnuts don't necessarily convey the message that the amount a nursing parent produces over a day rises rapidly in the first 10 days or so and if all is going well volumes produced can increase from 1oz on Day 1 to an incredible 20oz on Day 7!

It is far, far better to concentrate on looking at your baby. Ask yourself if he's gaining weight, appears happy and healthy and has a good nappy output. This is much more important than getting hooked up on images and figures.

The first milk you produce is called Colostrum and then anywhere from day 2-5 you will produce mature milk. Colostrum is thicker and more yellow than mature milk and is like your baby's first immunisation as it is highly concentrated and full of antibodies.

It is very important to allow a baby to feed whenever they signal for it because milk is made on a supply and demand basis. So, the more a baby feeds at the breast the more milk will be made. As baby suckles Prolactin and Oyxtocin are released making and ejecting the milk. Limiting time at the breast will signal to the body that baby does not require milk so less will be made- chemical messengers called Feedback Inhibitor of Lactation (FIL) will be released halting milk production.

Dee Bell, (Lactation Consultant, Midwife and Tongue Tie Practitioner) states *'The baby should be skin-to-skin with the nursing parent as much as possible during the first 3 days (and beyond). Research shows that this contact has a large impact on the mothering hormones of Prolactin and Oxytocin and the activation of the Acini cells (the milk-making cells). In the first 3 days, the baby should be skin-to-skin with the nursing parent whenever they are awake, as this is vital to encourage feeding and also to calm the baby. If other members of the family want to hold the baby, this is best done when the baby is asleep and will enable the birthing parent to rest.'*

How else can you help your baby attach to the breast effectively?

Firstly, it is important to be as relaxed as possible so that lots of Oxytocin is flowing to help expel the milk, supporting yourself with cushions behind your back so that you are comfortable and your shoulders are relaxed. Being skin to skin with baby will help initiate his inbuilt reflexes of touch, smell and taste to latch successfully. Also don't forget to have a drink of water to hand as breastfeeding is thirsty work! It is the mother who does the positioning and the baby who does the attachment. The way the baby approaches the breast and nipple is important for a good attachment. The nipple needs to be pointing up towards the baby's nostrils and then the baby is able to take a really big mouthful of breast tissue:

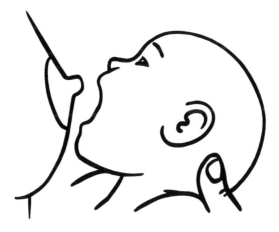

The nipple does not need to go square into the baby's mouth as this means the nipple points towards the throat and gets squashed by the hard palate causing pain for the mother and poor milk transfer:

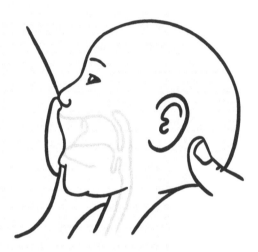

The baby needs to be tucked in close and tight to the nursing person so there is no space between baby's chest and parent's chest. By allowing the breast to sit naturally, adjusting the baby's body position in relation to the nipple, the baby approaches the breast with their chin making contact first and the baby's bottom lip a long way from the base of the nipple. The nipple will be pointing up towards the nostrils which allows him to take a really big mouthful of breast tissue, with the nipple just folding into the top of the mouth reaching the soft palate at the back:

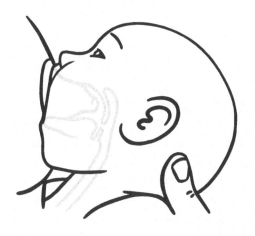

The baby's chin should be well off the baby's chest, with his head tipped back as he reaches up for the nipple. The baby will have a double chin! Signs that the baby is attached effectively are that his chin is indented into the breast allowing the chin to massage the breast tissue, his mouth will be open really wide with his top lip gently turned to face the breast, his nose will be free and his cheeks will appear rounded and full.

Note that we don't need to look for the bottom lip being turned outwards as this could disturb the latch. If the latch feels right, it is right so leave it alone! There will be more areola visible above the baby's top lip, whatever position he may be in. Finally, take off mitts and hats as the baby needs to be able to use all his senses to find the breast and feed whilst you breathe in his gorgeous newborn scent!

5 principles of good positioning for every feeding posture are:

- Baby's knees, hips, shoulders and cheeks all in line.
- Nipple pointing up nostrils.
- Head free to tilt back- baby can reach up to breast – nipple to soft palate and baby takes a deep mouthful of breast.
- Baby's body is supported, held close against Mum's body- no space.
- Posture is sustainable.

A baby who is ineffectively attached to the breast can lead to:

- Sore/damaged/cracked nipples.
- Engorgement leading to Mastitis- the breast is not being drained well so there is milk left behind, breasts are full and can become inflamed.
- Low milk supply as breasts aren't producing enough because milk transfer is poor so the demand isn't there.
- Slow/poor weight gain due to ineffective milk transfer.
- Jaundice due to extra milk not there to flush out the red blood cells.
- Hypernatremia- effects baby's sodium levels and electrolytes so baby becomes dehydrated which can lead to kidney failure.

There are a number of positions you can hold baby in to feed. I suggest avoiding the cradle hold in the first couple of months. This is where you support the baby with the arm on the same side as the nursing breast. Firstly, the cradle hold often puts baby at the wrong position to attach to the breast. They can come too far past the breast meaning that the baby comes down onto the nipple rather than reaching up to it. This is what causes a painful latch and ineffective milk transfer. Also, if baby isn't tucked in well there will be a gap between mother and baby.

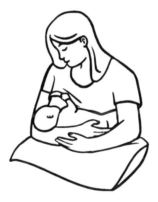

Cross cradle hold

This position is good for the early weeks as it achieves a more effective attachment. It puts the baby at a better position to effectively attach as the baby is close and secure to Mum, his bottom is tucked in and the baby is at a diagonal. He is reaching up to the breast, chin leading with the nipple pointing up the nostrils.

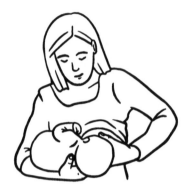

1. Phone, remote and a drink to hand!

2. Bring baby's bottom up towards your rib cage and use the opposite arm to the side you're feeding off to support the nape of the baby's neck.

3. The baby will come up towards the breast. Bottom tucked into you, legs wrapped around, chin makes contact first. Nipple points towards baby's nostrils.

4. Your palm is facing up to the sky rather than into your body.

5. Baby's feet should be together and not separated by your arm.

6. You can use your free arm to shape the breast. Don't pick the breast up! (More on breast shaping later on in this chapter).

7. There shouldn't be any space between your body and your baby's.

8. Your spare hand can support your opposite wrist not whole arm as this tucks baby in. Baby's head needs to be able to tip backwards when necessary.

9. You can then lean back slightly if necessary for your comfort.

Rugby ball hold

So called because baby is held like a rugby ball under the arm and tucked in close! Good for all body shapes but particularly those whose nipples point down as the baby comes up to the breast. Also helpful for a c-section as baby is nowhere near the area. Helps if nipples are sore as it ensures the nipple is up the nose, not pointing directly into the mouth, aiding a deeper latch. Also brings baby in close so they feel secure. Useful for feeding twins.

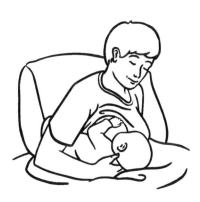

1. Phone, remote and a drink to hand!

2. Place a pillow lengthways behind your back and shuffle forwards on the seat leaving enough room for your elbows to run backwards whilst still tucked in close to your body.

3. Place another pillow under the arm of the side you're feeding from- not placed too high- baby needs to come UP to the breast from underneath.

4. Bring baby onto the side you're feeding from and bring her all the way back so her nose is opposite your nipple. Her feet may well touch the back of the sofa!

5. Your hand supports baby's neck, and your palm should be facing your face.

6. Baby looking at your opposite shoulder.

7. Baby's arm under your breast. Other arm over top. Both mitt free!

8. No gap between bodies. Chest to breast. Mum's elbow tucked in.

9. Chin to breast first. Nipple UP nostrils.

10. Other hand for breast shaping. Don't lift the breast.

11. Then place a rolled up towel underneath your wrist for support (NOT underneath baby as this will disturb the latch).

12. Repeat on other side.

Biological nurturing/Laid back feeding

Baby led as it initiates baby's innate reflexes to breastfeed. Good if baby has an ineffective attachment and Mum is sore. Can be used any time, day or night. It allows Mum to rest and relax. Useful for feeding twins. Useful for baby with colic/reflux. Can also bottle feed this way.

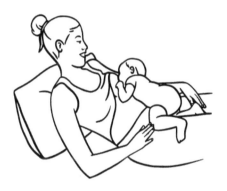

1. Have the remote, phone and some water to hand. You can be skin to skin if you like.

2. Lay back, ensuring you are sitting on your sacrum not your coccyx. Ensure your back, shoulders and nape of the neck are supported for a sustainable amount of time.

3. Bring baby in for a cuddle facing your cleavage, ensuring his feet and knees are attached to you so he can use them to crawl up towards the breast using those inbuilt reflexes. This pummelling action stimulates uterine contractions to help the uterus return to its original size.

4. Check his arms and hands are free as he will need to use these to find the breast and cuddle you. You'll notice at this stage how strong his neck muscles are as he begins to bob about lifting his head up!

5. Allow him to find the breast in his own time. Don't rush the process. Remember he is using his innate reflexes to find the breast and feed.

6. Shape the breast if necessary to help baby latch.

7. You can put an arm down the side to make sure he doesn't fall and use the other arm to stroke his back or for breast compressions!

8. Take a deep breath and consciously relax shoulders into the cushions!

Other benefits of this position are that you can inhale that gorgeous newborn smell from your baby's head, you're more likely to be in tune with your baby's feeding cues and it eases pressure off your perineum, allowing it to air and heal. You can also feed a bottle-fed baby in the biological nurturing position too!

Side-lying feeding

This position is really helpful to allow you to rest whilst you feed but also if you're recovering from a caesarean section or episiotomy.

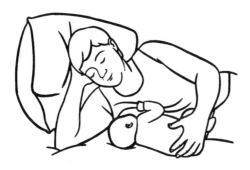

1. Lie on your side facing your baby and support your neck with a pillow (ensuring its well away from baby) and bend your knees. The arm you're lying on can lie along the bed outstretched, parallel with the top of baby's head. This gives him the freedom to tip his head back.
2. Bring baby to you and roll him onto his side so your nipple is level with his nose.
3. Ensure baby comes to the breast chin leading and mouth wide open.
4. You may find it more comfortable to place a rolled up blanket or towel between your knees to ease pressure on your back.

How do we know baby is getting enough milk?

Good positioning from the nursing parent allows effective attachment for the baby which leads to effective milk transfer. Parents need to look out for signs that the baby is hungry and feed, feed, feed! The baby cups the nipple and breast tissue with his tongue. The jaw lowers and a vacuum is created which draws the milk in. The baby then closes his mouth- the jaw and tongue move up which closes the ducts. When the mouth is full of milk the baby swallows. The main signs of effective milk transfer are the baby's sucks and swallows. These will change throughout the course of a typical feed. The baby will begin with call up, short sucks and lots of rapid swallows (1:1) as the let-down reflex happens. He will then begin active feeding where there are longer, slower, more rhythmical sucks with swallows, then pauses, along with maybe two or three further let downs (2/3:1 interspersed with 1:1). Finally, the baby may 'flutter suck' at the end of a feed where they'll suck with fewer swallows before usually falling asleep. (Please do go and check out the suck and swallow videos online- lots of Lactation Consultants have these on their Instagram pages- I promise knowing the difference between a suck and a swallow will make all the difference!)

Baby will have his chin firmly touching the breast, his mouth will be wide open and nose free, more of the areola will be visible above baby's top lip, his cheeks will be rounded, Mum won't feel pain, Mum will hear when baby swallows (a 'kuh' sound as air passes through the nose) or see the jaw drop, and baby will be happy and content between feeds.

Babies will generally feed 8-12 times in 24 hours and if they're not signalling for it we are looking for feeds 3 hourly from the start of one feed to the start of the next (it's always a good idea to offer both sides). Once baby is well past her birth weight, is gaining weight well, has a good nappy output and is fit and well then we can follow her lead at night.

The baby will commonly have poo which changes from Meconium (Marmite) to changing stool (Pesto) to mustard yellow (Korma) thereafter twice a day with 6 wet nappies.

With regards to weight, we are looking at whether baby has regained his birth weight by 2 weeks (thereafter gaining 30-40g per day in the first three months and an average of 20g per day between 3 and 6 months, as suggested by WHO). Is he tracking close to his centile? Is baby settled between feeds? Is he healthy and alert when awake and calm/relaxed when breastfeeding?

Breast shaping

Something else you can try to aid a deeper latch is to shape the breast before your baby latches. This enables baby to take a larger amount of breast tissue into his mouth and can be helpful if you have large breasts or baby seems to be slipping off as he feeds. How you shape the breast is key though. Think of it as taking a bite from a sandwich. You wouldn't take a bite of a sandwich with it held vertically as there would be too much surface area for you to get your mouth around. Instead, we hold the sandwich horizontally so we can take a good-sized bite. It's exactly the same when we shape the breast for baby to attach. Depending on which way you have positioned baby will depend on how you shape the breast though, generally speaking in either a C or a U shape. The best way to remember this is to always have your thumb parallel to baby's top lip, that way you know you're shaping in the correct way to suit baby's position. So, in a biological nurturing position you'd use the C shape and the cross cradle hold you'd use the U shape. You need to create a U or a C shape with your thumb and index finger placed behind the areola so you don't affect the latch. Squeeze together and wait for baby to attach.

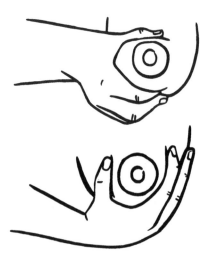

Breast compressions

This involves applying pressure to the breast with the opposite hand to the side you're feeding off to help continue the flow of milk. This is a really useful tool if you have a sleepy baby at the breast, or you have a baby who is keen on the faster flow of a let-down, perhaps they're struggling with slow weight gain or when you're pumping and trying to increase milk output. You can simply place the palm of your hand over the top of the breast and apply pressure or put your hand around the breast in a c shape and squeeze towards the chest wall where the milk making cells are, holding for a long slow squeeze. When baby stops swallowing you can release. Repeat as required.

My breasts feel empty, help!

Your breasts are never truly empty. Milk production is ongoing and the more breastmilk baby takes the more your body makes, it's like a factory! Your breasts may feel emptier towards the end of the day but this is entirely normal and as long as your baby is happy, healthy, gaining weight and has a good nappy output then there is nothing to be concerned about.

My baby is very fussy in the evenings. What is cluster feeding?

This is very common and normal in the early months. Your baby might feed, fuss, cry and then feed, fuss and cry again which may go on for some time. This can be a prime time for your confidence in your body's ability to nourish your baby to drop and many parents worry they aren't producing enough milk and so revert to a bottle just in case. However, giving your baby a bottle will signal to your body to halt production and make less milk. Formula fed babies have fussy evenings too. Ensure you have snacks, the tv remote and your phone at hand during these tough times. Remember that your baby will be getting a higher fat concentration of milk at this time of the day and if they appear fussy due to a slower flow of milk then some breast compressions may help. One reason for babies being particularly fussy at this time of day is perhaps due to overstimulation and the day spent adjusting to their new world. They wish to seek comfort in the form of you, their home. You could try carrying, taking a bath together, some baby massage, a walk or some white noise. Having someone there not only as an extra pair of hands but to listen to you is really important, if at all possible.

What about fore and hind milk?

Many so-called experts believe the breasts produce two distinct types of milk, fore milk (watery) and hind milk (fatty). However, this is not the case! As breastmilk is made, the fatty milk stays higher in the breast sticking to the milk ducts, whilst the more watery milk moves towards the nipple to mix with the fattier milk left there from the previous feed. The fuller the breast/the longer the time between feeds, the more diluted this leftover milk will become. As long as breastfeeding is going well then allow baby to feed when he wants and he will receive enough fat.

Do I need to take any supplements when I breastfeed?

The NHS website states *'It's recommended that breastfed babies are given a daily supplement containing 8.5 to 10 micrograms of Vitamin D from birth, whether or not you're taking a supplement containing Vitamin D yourself.'*

Practises that can interfere with breastfeeding

- Disturbing the newborn's nine instinctive behaviours- baby then has to go back to step one and imprinting, in which baby learns to recognise his mother, is lost.
- Dummy- baby's hunger cues can be missed.

- Formula- if a baby has formula then he won't be feeding from the breast so the demand will reduce, in turn reducing milk supply. Breast milk supply needs to be protected in this instance.
- Offering a bottle that isn't pace fed- baby gets used to a faster flow of milk (more on paced feeding later).
- Not keeping mother and baby together- parents aren't as able to pick up on baby's feeding cues and unlimited access to the breast is lost.
- Breastfeeding pillow- as discussed earlier a baby should come to the breast with their chin leading and their head tipped back. Placing a pillow on your lap may position baby too high, causing her to come to the breast at the wrong angle, leading to a shallow latch. The pillow might also encourage you to move the breast towards baby's mouth rather than allowing the breast to sit naturally. It is far better to position yourself and allow baby to attach first, and then bring in pillows afterwards for support where needed. NB However, a correctly fitted breastfeeding pillow for twins may be useful!
- Routine- keeping baby on a strict feeding schedule can negatively impact milk supply as the breasts aren't receiving the signal to produce more milk, Feedback Inhibitor of Lactation is released and milk production slows.
- Some parents may be keeping to one breast per feed because they have been told that they need to

keep baby on one side for long enough to reach the hind milk. This is out of date advice and can affect supply because the other breast is not being stimulated.

- Swaddling- A study published by BASIS in February 2023 found that *'Infants swaddled immediately after birth show a delay in initial breastfeeding, less successful suckling at the breast, reduced intake of breastmilk and greater weight loss compared to un-swaddled babies. Swaddling visually obscures feeding cues and reduces crying, thereby eliminating two key feeding prompts typically used by parents/carers.'*

Expressing

As a Breastfeeding Counsellor I can support parents with pumping for an occasional bottle, i.e. if you are going to be apart from your baby for a short time because you might need to go to the dentist or an appointment. If, however, you're needing to pump to increase milk supply, if your baby is not gaining sufficient weight, or if you're returning to work and are therefore going to be away from your baby for a longer period of time then I would always signpost to a Lactation Consultant.

Firstly, if all is going well for you and your baby and there are no health concerns then there is no need to pump between feeds to make more milk in the early weeks. I have heard of others recommending this to parents as a sort of insurance policy for future milk supply, but the risk here is that you could end up with an oversupply issue which can lead to issues such as Engorgement, Mastitis and a baby with green frothy poos. Your baby and body need time to get in sync with one another, after all your body doesn't know if you've had one baby, two or more, so let your baby be the guide! However, clearly if you're separated from your baby or your baby is struggling to latch then you need to maintain your milk supply and hand expressing colostrum and pumping mature milk will be key.

Your choices for expressing are to hand express, use a manual pump (a pump operated by your hand), a hospital grade pump (very strong and good for increasing supply) or an electric pump (operated by battery or power outlet, single or double).

Hand expressing can be more effective than a pump in the early days when colostrum is thick and breasts may be swollen. Colostrum can get stuck in a pump and we don't want to lose ANY of this liquid gold. Hand expressing reduces the chance of cross contamination as there is no equipment required and it may elicit a more effective hormonal response than a pump, yielding more milk. You can also hand express before, during and after manual pumping to help increase the calorific content of the milk and aid more milk removal, in turn stimulating production.

If you're using a manual or electric pump it is important that you find one that fits correctly. The flange which is the piece of the breast pump that fits over your breast needs to be secure enough that there is a seal but not so tight that it leaves a mark and blocks the milk ducts. You will need to measure the diameter of your nipple also to make sure that the flange is the correct size- too big and the pump can't milk the breast properly as there will be an air vacuum and too small means the nipple will rub against the pump and make you sore. Check with the manufacturer of the pump.

Begin by warming up/massaging the breast. When you turn on an electric pump it will start by mimicking the baby sucking and the pump will work quite fast, stimulating a spike in hormones to release the milk. Once you notice drops of milk starting to appear you can switch the pump to the next mode which will slow down the pump action to mimic sucks and swallows. You can compress the breast during this time to help contract the milk ducts and expel the milk but keep your hands away from the flange so you don't affect the suction. Some pumps have varying speeds but it is best to set yours to a comfortable setting- you won't yield more milk just by turning the pump up to maximum speed, often this can have the opposite effect. You may choose to express whilst feeding your baby from the other side as baby will stimulate a let-down and Oxytocin will be higher at this time.

If you wish to pump to allow someone else to give a bottle or if you need to leave your baby to attend an appointment then either pump 2-3 times the day before (pumping routinely will increase supply which you don't want if you're pumping as a one off) or about 30-45 minutes after the first feed of the day as milk is more abundant at this time, for no longer than about 20 minutes. Olivia Hinge, Lactation Consultant and NHS Midwife has a fabulous Instagram account @olivia_lactation_consultant where she states that *'We are expecting 30-40mls per hour that you're apart from your baby. We don't really want to be giving a breastfed baby more than 120-150mls of milk in one sitting because they probably wouldn't receive more than that from the breast, so little and often is the best way to do this... Then after those 8 weeks you suddenly start to find actually whenever you pump you're only getting 10-20mls each boob- totally, totally normal! Your body is so clever that it makes exactly the right amount of milk for your baby for them to grow well, do enough wees and poos a day, not to stock up your freezer at slightly unpredictable times as well... For most people you would have to be doing 2 or 3 pump sessions in a day to get a substantial volume for one bottle feed.'*

As Olivia says, you may find that once your milk supply is established the amount you pump decreases. As long as baby is gaining weight and has plenty of wet and dirty nappies then this is normal. Your body is incredible and makes exactly what your baby requires. The tricky thing with expressing is it can make us feel very anxious about amounts, something which we were oblivious to before the pump was brought in.

Don't be alarmed if your baby takes little or no milk whilst you're gone. The caregiver could try offering your milk in a cup/syringe/spoon instead or wearing a muslin that smells of you (ensure used milk is discarded within 1-2 hours). Your baby might just go on a nursing strike whilst you're away and feed, feed, feed on your return!

Parts of the pump may need to be replaced every few months, such as the valve and membrane which create the suction. These look like bumpy, white, thin bits of plastic inside the pump.

Pumping to increase supply

I held a Q&A session with the wonderful Hannah Croft. Hannah and I have been friends for almost 20 years and trained together at Norland College. Hannah is now an International Board Certified Lactation Consultant based in Kent and lives with her husband and two children. She has a private practice and works for a digital health company and the NHS.

Q. What are the signs that my milk supply is low?

A. Signs of low milk supply may include;
- having breasts that did not change during pregnancy; no increase in size or change in nipple/areola size and colour.

- having a baby who feeds very frequently, who seems unsettled, and who has few wet and dirty nappies, and may struggle to gain weight appropriately.
- not seeing an increase in milk volume when pumping, or using techniques like compressions and switch nursing to increase the volumes produced.

It's really important to work with an IBCLC to determine that feeding is optimised as much as possible. If baby's positioning and attachment to the breast isn't great, this could impact milk removal and thus impact the feedback system to make more milk. An IBCLC will also take a full medical history to ascertain anything that may indicate markers for low milk supply.

Q. What causes low milk supply?

A. There are many factors which may contribute to or cause low milk supply. Some can be reversed, others not.

- Poor breastfeeding management-separation of mother and baby, scheduling or limiting feeds, keeping baby on one breast per feed rather than watching for signs of swallowing.
- Poor breast attachment- if milk is not adequately removed from the breast this may reduce breastmilk supply.
- Breast anatomy; insufficient glandular tissue (IGT) can mean that it's not possible to make a full supply. There are some physical markers for this including widely spaced, or tubular breasts, but we can't always tell just from looking.

- A baby who is not able to feed effectively; maybe due to low weight gain, or anatomical issues like torticollis or tongue-tie.
- Hormone or endocrine issues- several hormones are required to make milk. If a mother has underlying hormonal issues or imbalances this could affect milk production.
- Breast surgery- any breast surgery including breast reduction or augmentation may impact the ability to make a full supply.
- Medications- some medications such as certain birth control, or even pain medications used in labour may reduce milk production.
- Retained placenta- any remnants of placenta left in the mother's uterus may mean milk supply is reduced.

Q. What can I do about it? How often do I pump, when and how long for? Will I ever be able to exclusively breastfeed again?

A. It's important to understand and recognise that ANY breastmilk you can give your baby is important and valuable. Breastfeeding doesn't have to be exclusive for it to count! That said, if you're keen to exclusively breastfeed there are ways you can try and achieve this. Understanding how milk is made, and removed is useful knowledge, and can help you feel empowered in your feeding experience.

If low milk supply is suspected, the first thing to do is to optimise feeding. This would include checking the latch of the baby and watching for signs of milk transfer. A baby with an effective suck and swallow is the best thing we have to boost supply! Increasing the amount of milk a baby is removing will drive the mother's supply so talk to an IBCLC about using breast compressions and switch nursing.

Sometimes using a breast pump can help boost milk supply too, particularly if the baby is unwell. The advantage of a breast pump is that it doesn't tire or get full like a baby!

Any pumping you can do will stimulate your supply, the more removed the more there will be. If you are exclusively pumping you ideally need to remove milk at least 8 times in 24 hours.

If baby is feeding directly as well, aim for a number of pumping sessions that feels sustainable rather than setting a target that feels impossible. If you do manage to squeeze in an extra session that day, great!

Try pumping after breastfeeds; an emptier breast will make milk faster and help ensure that your breast is effectively drained. Lots of mums have success first thing in the morning, and then see volumes lower as the day goes on, this is ok and can be normal!

It's better to do more frequent, shorter pumping sessions, rather than less frequent longer ones. Use the pump until the milk flow stops, usually 10-15 mins per breast is about right, but if the milk keeps flowing, keep going! Use hands on pumping to squeeze, stroke and massage the breasts during pumping.

Think about supplementing your baby at the breast. Speak to an IBCLC about using an at breast supplementer, rather than using a bottle. This way, your baby continues to feed at the breast, and your breasts get that extra stimulation to try and increase supply.

Sometimes families are put on a plan of 'triple feeding.' This involves feeding at the breast, pumping and supplementing the baby with either expressed breastmilk (EBM) or formula. A plan like this should only really be used short term as it is exhausting and intense. If you're not seeing the changes you'd like to after a few days, go back to your healthcare provider and see if you can adjust the plan to make it more sustainable.

Q. Do you have any tips for choosing a pump?

A. Not all pumps are equal! If you are thinking about using a pump, consider how you're planning to use it, and think about your budget too. Buy the best you can afford and go for a reputable brand.

If it is to boost your supply it may be worth considering renting a pump; these are usually the sort used in hospital with a strong, powerful motor designed to stimulate the breasts in the absence of a baby there to do it.

Try and avoid second-hand pumps, especially those with an 'open system'. They are not designed to be multi-user pumps, and over time the motors degenerate which will impact the milk removal, and therefore potentially your supply.

Silicone pumps have grown in popularity, like the 'Haakaa'. They are easy to use and clean, and very portable. They collect the let-down of the breast not being used. However, some caution is needed with these as they can cause oversupply.

Q. Any tips for pumping?

A. Pumping is a different ballgame to breastfeeding and it can take a bit of time to perfect the skill so don't be disheartened if you don't get loads of milk out straight away.

Try having your baby near you when you pump so you can utilise the oxytocin. An item of their clothing you can sniff or a photo might work too.

Have some relaxing music on, or something funny on the tv or radio. Get those happy, relaxed hormones flowing.

On the same note, it's been shown that orgasm can help with pumping; again, all that Oxytocin has a positive effect!

Try warming the flanges (the bits that touch your breast) before you pump. Run through with warm water before you start.

Use your hands to gently massage and compress your

breasts while you pump. Google 'hands on pumping' for more information on this. Research has shown it can help get up to 50% more milk out!

Although the NHS say to sterilise pump parts after every time, in the US the advice is (as long as your baby is full term, and healthy) to simply do a hot, soapy wash of pump parts between uses. Some families even choose to store pump parts in the fridge between uses to save time too.

Pumping shouldn't hurt, do check the flanges fit appropriately too. You want your nipple to move fairly freely in the flange, but not too much areola to be sucked in.

Consider doing some power pumping. This is a technique used to mimic cluster feeding, and the idea is that you do short, frequent bursts of pumping. Pick an hour of the day, and do 10 minutes of pumping, then 10 minutes break, then alternate for the rest of the time period. For some mums this can be an effective and helpful tool to boost supply in a time efficient way.

It's fine to combine and use milk from different pumping sessions. It's best to mix them once they're at the same temperature.

Combination/mixed feeding (by choice not necessity)

It is advised that a bottle isn't introduced in the first six weeks to allow breastfeeding to become established. From this stage some parents wish to introduce the odd bottle of formula. This doesn't have to mean the end of your breastfeeding journey if you don't want it to. However, remember that the less milk baby takes from the breast the less the breast makes, so by introducing bottles of formula you are signalling to your body to slow down production. You may be happy for your supply to decrease and gradually be replaced with formula and in this instance if you feel full when the bottle is given then hand expressing to comfort will help. However, if you're planning on formula feeding temporarily then you will need to consider expressing when the formula is given to signal to your body to continue making milk.

It is crucial when bottle feeding to pace feed so that the breastfeeding relationship is protected and baby doesn't get used to a faster flow of milk and a different way of feeding, leading to frustration at the breast and potentially rejection.

The key is to mimic your baby's breastfeeding pattern as closely as possible by feeding responsively. Follow his hunger cues and never force him to finish a bottle. Remember that breasts don't have a gauge, so we never know exactly how much milk a baby has taken, instead we look at other signs that they're having enough. Bottle feeding should be the same- try not to be tempted to make up a set amount of formula and stress if the baby leaves some. We want baby to feed according to their appetite and to assess when they're full. It is always better to make up a small feed and then make a little more if he signals for it. Trust baby not the tin!

Milk banks and milk sharing sites

Milk from a UK milk bank has been screened and pasteurised. However, milk from a milk sharing site has not, so it can include transmission of certain infections (from an asymptomatic mother), medicines, drugs or environmental contaminants due to poor hygiene when handling and storing the milk.

When a woman offers her breastmilk to a milk bank she is asked if she smokes, drinks regularly or uses recreational drugs. She is also asked if she has tested positive for certain diseases including Hepatitis. She is asked about the health of her and her baby, if she has been exposed to any harmful chemicals or if she has had any recent medical intervention i.e. exposure to radiotherapy. If she answers yes to any of the above then she cannot donate milk. If she is successful then her milk is screened for HIV 1 and 2, Hepatitis B and C, HTLV I and II, and Syphilis.

In comparison milk sharing sites do not ask you to complete any of these checks so a baby who receives such milk is potentially put at risk.

Banked milk is prioritised for sick and premature babies in hospital. If there is enough banked milk then it is made available to parents facing challenges. A healthcare professional is required to oversee the process to ensure the milk is being used appropriately and to give additional support to Mum.

Storing Colostrum and mature milk

When storing colostrum it may split and appear to have frozen in two halves. You may notice an orange colour to it which is the fat, and some might be tinged with red which is bleeding from the capillaries (this is normal so don't be alarmed). Freeze syringes within 24 hours.

To store unused mature milk the following is recommended:

Four hours @ room temperature (3 hours on hot days).

Four days in the fridge @ the back, below 4°c.

Six months in the freezer (2 weeks in an ice compartment, 12 months in a chest freezer).

It is sensible to freeze milk in small quantities to avoid waste.

Common problems

Engorgement

This is when your breasts feel overly full and swollen with milk. This can be normal when your milk first 'comes in' as extra fluids and blood will be in the breast to help with production. Also, if your baby has slept longer than usual between feeds, baby is ineffectively attached to the breast or you're feeding on a schedule rather than on demand then the breasts may feel engorged. If engorged breasts are left untreated then Mastitis can develop. Keeping baby close, skin to skin, so that she has unlimited access to the breast (feeding min 8-12 times in 24 hours) can help, hand expressing to comfort, as well as a technique called Reverse Pressure Softening which helps drain fluid away from the area to allow baby to latch. You can do this by creating a flower shape around the base of the nipple with your fingertips and pushing back towards the chest wall, counting slowly to 50. The pressure should be firm but not painful. Repeat this process until the area has softened. If you're excessively engorged then lying on your back to do this may help further. Maya Bolman IBCLC also talks about 'breast gymnastics' where you massage the breast in such a way that any fluid drains back into the lymphatic system. Some women find relief from cold savoy cabbage leaves from the fridge placed in their bra between feeds as these shrink the blood vessels in the breast, reducing swelling and pain, however care must be taken to stop using these after swelling has reduced as they can negatively impact your supply.

Blocked ducts

Your breast may feel hard, lumpy and tender to touch. Unlike with Mastitis you should still feel well in yourself. A blocked duct is due to excess milk causing inflammation of the breast tissue that then surrounds and compresses the milk ducts. Causes may be ineffective attachment, tight fitting clothing, missed feeds or previous breast surgery. Seek support for positioning and attachment, feed at least 8-12 times in 24 hours, use cold therapy, try gentle breast massage towards the lymph nodes in the armpits and be guided by baby before moving him to the other breast to feed. It is important not to over pump as this can lead to an oversupply and make the problem worse.

Mastitis

Mastitis comes under the umbrella of breast inflammation and just like with a blocked duct is thought to be caused by a build-up of milk within the ducts of the breast. It can lead to a very sore, red or darkened breast and can cause flu-like symptoms.

The build-up of milk and inflammation can be related to oversupply, poor positioning and attachment (including from a breast pump), a baby who is fed to a schedule or where breastfeeding is stopped abruptly, pressure on the breast (e.g. from a tight-fitting bra, breast trauma or vigorous massage), a history of Mastitis, smoking, stress, an imbalance of the microbiome within the body due to poor diet or a bacterial infection caused by Staphylococcus Aureus or Streptococcus.

In the past nursing parents were told to feed, feed, feed, apply heat and massage the breast to help clear the inflammation. If, for example, oversupply is the root cause you can see why the feed, feed, feed message would do more harm than good here.

In June 2022 The Academy of Breastfeeding Medicine suggested the following treatment instead:

- Optimising positioning and attachment, seeking help from a Lactation Consultant where possible.
- Feeding baby on demand, but where this isn't possible hand expressing to comfort, NOT to 'empty' the breast as this can perpetuate the issue of oversupply. Remember that it is normal for babies to feed 8-12 times in 24 hours.
- Give the breast a spa day, applying only the same pressure as you would to stroke a pet. You can try some 'breast gymnastics' where you move the breast gently in circular motions between the palm of your hands.
- Double check you have a correctly fitted nursing bra.

- Consume a well-balanced diet and drink plenty of fluids.
- Seek help to ensure your breast pump flange fits you correctly.
- Avoid applying heat as this can exacerbate inflammation by causing blood vessels to dilate! A cold compress applied for about 20 minutes is best. Alternatively, savoy cabbage leaves that have been kept in the fridge can be worn in your bra.
- The website breastfeeding.support states the following about pain relief: *'Compatible pain-killers or anti-inflammatory medication may help mothers cope with pain and inflammation (ABM 2022). Ibuprofen and paracetamol are compatible with breastfeeding. However, Douglas points out that over reliance on medications to bring down a fever can interfere with the body's own mechanisms to down regulate the inflammatory response (Douglas, Vol 18:1-20 2022).'*.
- The guidelines for antibiotics are that if the nursing person doesn't feel better within 12-24 hours or is very unwell then to seek medical attention, but that antibiotics are only for bacterial Mastitis and for a 10-14 day course. If used incorrectly for inflammatory Mastitis they can disrupt the microbiome which can lead on to bacterial Mastitis. The Academy of Breastfeeding Medicine also states; *'Prophylactic antibiotics have not been shown to be effective in the*

prevention of Mastitis. It should be noted that many antibiotics and antifungal medications have anti-inflammatory properties, and this may explain why women experience relief when taking these.'.

Pain

If your baby is correctly attached to the breast you shouldn't feel any pain. If you have sore, cracked or damaged nipples then please seek support from an IBCLC or Breastfeeding Counsellor. In the meantime, you'll need to protect your milk supply by hand expressing (at any stage of breastfeeding) or using a pump (once your milk comes in, but ensure the pump fits you correctly). You can use breastmilk on the nipple to aid healing and counter infection. Moist wound healing is advised but some people can be allergic to lanolin-based nipple creams and due to their high grease content babies can slip off the breast. Lanolin free nipple creams might therefore be more suitable, or alternatively a hydrogel pad. Ensure you wash your hands before applying and change breast pads regularly. The laid-back feeding position is also worth a try to help achieve a deeper latch. If you need to unlatch baby before trying a new position due to pain, then gently slide your little finger into the corner of his mouth to break the suction.

Lipstick nipple

If, when your baby finishes a feed, your nipple looks lipstick shaped then this is a sign that the nipple is being pressed against the hard palate, so positioning and attachment needs to be looked at.

Thrush

Thrush is caused by a type of Candida yeast that lives naturally on our bodies, common areas being the mouth and groin. Your areola or nipple may feel itchy, red, cracked and appear flakey or shiny. Typically, both nipples will be affected as baby feeds off both. You may experience a sharp stabbing feeling deep within the breast as a feed progresses or after a feed and this can come on suddenly. You may like to consider booking an appointment with a breastfeeding specialist to double check positioning and attachment first, as this could in fact be the root cause of the pain and unnecessary treatment can be avoided. Thrush is very often misdiagnosed and can in fact be Vasospasm (discussed shortly) or a bacterial infection and the latter of the two can only be confirmed with a swab taken by the GP. If your baby does have thrush, he may display symptoms such as raised white lesions on the tongue and the insides of the cheeks (like cottage cheese), nappy rash and redness/irritation around the lips. However, it is possible for your baby not to have any symptoms. It is important to keep feeding through thrush and to seek medical advice from your GP. Both you and your baby will need to be treated and you must take care to ensure you wash your hands, feeding equipment and clothes regularly.

Baby not latching

This can be affected by type of delivery, if baby was premature (or before 39 weeks and small), unwell or you were separated from one another. You may need to supplement your baby with milk you've expressed, donor milk or formula (by bottle/cup/finger feeding). Your main priority if baby isn't latching is to protect your supply and keep baby fed. Ensure you express a minimum of 8-10 times in 24 hours, with no longer than one six-hour gap between, and feed this to baby (hand expressing colostrum and using an electric pump when your mature milk comes in). Parents used to be advised to include at least one pumping session at night due to Prolactin levels being highest at this point, however, a study conducted by Dr Ilana Levene from the John Radcliffe Hospital in Oxford in 2022 showed Prolactin levels actually peak more gently overnight and that expressing overnight didn't lead to a greater overall yield. You could give your baby a syringe of colostrum expressed antenatally- this might give her the boost of energy she needs to come to the breast. Plenty of skin to skin, laid back feeding to stimulate baby's natural inbuilt reflexes to feed, expressing a bit of milk out onto the nipples to entice baby to feed, wearing your baby in a sling, taking a bath together or seeking the help of a Lactation Consultant to help you use a nursing supplementer. This is a piece of tubing that slides into the corner of baby's mouth and the other end is placed into a bottle of milk. As baby feeds at the breast, they are rewarded with milk from the bottle whilst also stimulating milk production with the aim being that they eventually feed independently at the breast.

Nipple Vasospasm

This can be caused by a shallow latch and affects blood supply and causes a sudden narrowing of the blood vessels. It has been connected to Raynaud's Phenomenon. You may feel pain in your breasts which worsens in the cold e.g. when exposing your nipple to feed or passing the refrigerator in the supermarket. You may also notice colour changes in your nipple after a feed and possibly have a history of circulation problems or migraines. Treatment includes optimizing the latch, not smoking and reducing caffeine as these constrict blood vessels, keeping nipples warm with a wheat bag, and avoiding decongestants/contraceptive pill/Fluconazole for thrush as these have been known to worsen symptoms.

Inverted nipples

This does not mean breastfeeding is impossible! Firstly, try breast stimulation as this may be enough to help the nipple become erect. The biological nurturing position can help as gravity aids your baby's latch and they're able to use those inbuilt reflexes. Similarly, you could try hand expressing or pumping for a short time before quickly whizzing baby onto the breast when the nipple is exposed. The breastfeeding.support website suggests *'Pulling back on the breast tissue as baby gapes to latch can help a nipple to protrude more (Mohrbacher, 2020 p739). The 'nipple nudge'- this involves pushing up into the breast through the areola and behind the nipple to help expose the nipple for the latch i.e. push it inside out.'* It is worth noting that some inverted nipples can become drawn out during a breastfeeding journey, as the tight tendons are torn. This can cause soreness around the nipples as the flesh is new and fresh. Moist wound healing will help with this.

Nipple shields

These are pieces of thin silicone that fit over your nipple and areola with a space cut out (depending on which way you wear it the space can either allow baby's nose to smell the breast or turned the other way creates a space for the tongue to make contact with the breast) and are often used on a nursing person with flat or inverted nipples to help baby latch. Firstly, it is recommended that in the early days nipple shields are avoided and that instead milk supply is protected and that unlimited skin to skin takes place so that those wonderful natural reflexes we discussed earlier are allowed to be exercised. If, once your milk comes in, you're still struggling then seeking support should be your first port of call. An IBCLC or breastfeeding specialist can check positioning and attachment first and, if following the tips above on inverted nipples hasn't helped, then ask about shields. The shield can help trigger a prem/sleepy baby's sucking reflex as the shield meets baby's palate, something which may be harder when feeding from flat/inverted nipples. Shields can also build a bridge between sore nipples and keeping the breastfeeding relationship going, however adjustment of the positioning and attachment may well be all it takes to ease discomfort without having to resort to shields. Sometimes shields can entice a baby back to the breast who has developed a preference for a bottle, but this is by no means the only solution. As always keep an eye on your baby's weight and nappy output to ensure they're getting enough milk if you are using shields. An ill-fitting shield can cause further problems so please seek help to find one that fits you correctly, it should not be painful.

Reflux

Carol Smyth a Lactation Consultant and CBT Psychotherapist from Northern Ireland has published a book called 'Why Infant Reflux Matters' which discusses the difference between Reflux and GORD- Gastro Oesophageal Reflux Disease. These are two different things. Babies with GORD tend to display symptoms such as sleep apnoea, a hoarse cry, ear infections, asthma or faltering growth despite a feeding assessment and treatment plan from a Lactation Consultant. The National Institute for Health & Care Excellence state that GORD should be investigated if two or more of these symptoms are present and this is usually done via an Endoscopy.

Reflux itself is considered to be normal in babies and the amount can vary from one baby to the next. As long as your baby is happy, healthy and gaining weight then this isn't normally a cause for concern. Some babies will exhibit posseting, so just a small amount of sick, whilst others will bring up whole feeds but aren't really bothered by this happening. And some reflux doesn't even reach baby's mouth at all!

Your baby's stomach is not like a ball, it is a J shaped organ with a valve at the top that goes off at a diagonal, and another valve at the bottom. As baby sucks the valve at the top opens to allow milk in. This valve remains open until baby's last swallow. Digestion then begins and the lower valve opens to allow the stomach contents to move into the intestines. There are a number of things that can cause this top valve to relax and open. These include trapped air, constipation, coughing, crying or when she's taken on a little too much milk. This is her body's way of expelling that extra food or gas! Some babies have a weaker valve than others which can lead to more spit up, however babies tend to settle within a few minutes, either wanting to feed again or just suck. Studies show reflux occurs in most babies due to their immature system. Many parents worry that they should be placing baby to sleep on an incline to help prevent reflux. Not only does this go against safer sleeping guidelines but studies show this makes no significant difference. Carol Smyth suggests looking at whether your baby is still unsettled or sick when they're on their back, whilst in your arms or on your body. If they are ok here then it suggests they just need to be with you, close to your body to sleep. A baby who is relaxed is less likely to have reflux as their sphincter muscle at the top of the stomach is tighter. Additionally, tummy time can also be beneficial to reflux as babies are designed to spend time on their tummies which puts them in a calmer state, again reducing reflux. Remember when placing a baby down to sleep not to put them down on their tummy though and to practice safer sleep guidelines. One final interesting fact to note is that newborns have very little stomach acid. In fact, acid levels rise in the first 3 weeks before declining between weeks 3 and 4, not reaching the levels of an adult until aged 3! The longer between the feeds the higher the levels of acid because milk neutralises this. Therefore, reflux is more likely when babies have larger more infrequent feeds.

Please seek a feeding assessment from a Lactation Consultant if you're at all worried.

Tongue Tie

(Q&A Session with IBCLC Hannah Croft)

Q. What is tongue tie?

A. We all have frenula all over our body, they are structures of tissue that hold mobile parts of our body together, including under our tongue.

A baby who appears to have a restrictive frenulum is said to be tongue tied. The medical name for this condition in ankyloglossia.

Until recently, it was thought that a tongue tie was a band, or stringy bit of tissue, but thanks to a study published in 2019, we now understand that it's more a fold of fascia, or tissue.

The position of the 'join' to the tongue can also vary its impact on feeding, as can the stretchiness of the tissue.

Q. How does tongue tie affect breastfeeding?

A. If the tongue's movement is restricted by a tight frenulum, then it may impact breastfeeding in several ways. These could include painful latch for the mother, leading to damaged nipples. It could also lead to ineffective milk removal leading to poor weight gain and unsettledness for the baby, and blocked ducts or mastitis for the mother, resulting in reduced milk supply.

According to the NICE guidelines there is some 'limited evidence' that dividing a tight, restrictive frenulum under the tongue may improve breastfeeding outcomes, particularly for maternal nipple pain.

Interestingly, at present, the NICE guidelines did not include this in their literature search when making their recommendations.

Q. How is a tongue tie assessed?

A. There isn't currently one single, agreed on, clinical tool for identifying a tongue tie, so this is an ongoing discussion within the feeding community. Because frenula are a normal, anatomical structure it can be difficult to differentiate between a normal lingual frenulum, and one that is restrictive.

The only practitioner able to officially diagnose a tongue tie is a Frenulotomist who is someone otherwise medically trained who has undergone specific training in tongue tie, but other practitioners can assess tongue function, and suggest that a tongue tie may be indicated.

It is important to examine function over form, so an examination is carried out by a trained practitioner using a gloved finger inside the baby's mouth, rather than simply looking in the baby's mouth. The practitioner is likely to investigate the tongue's ability to lateralise (move from side to side), extend (protrude over the bottom lip), elevate (be able to reach mid-way in the mouth when the mouth is open, and cup (seal to the breast or teat.) The practitioner will also note the shape of the baby's palate, and how the movement of the tongue feels when the baby sucks. Finally, they will sweep under the tongue to feel for any possible restriction.

Q. Does it always need a frenulotomy?

A. A frenulotomy is the name for the procedure to divide the tongue tie.
Just because a frenulum is visible, or palpable, it does not mean that it needs to be divided.

Research in 2002 found an incidence of 10.8% babies with tongue tie, with only 50% of those actually requiring a division.

This is why skilled breastfeeding support is always the first port of call with feeding issues. Although a frenulotomy is a low-risk procedure, we do want to avoid babies undergoing the surgery unless it is truly necessary. Often many of the issues experienced during breastfeeding can be rectified with improving positioning, latching, and milk removal.

If a frenulotomy is required, it is likely that the feeding dyad will need feeding support before and after the procedure to help get feeding back on track.
Frenulotomy is certainly not a 'quick fix' and skilled, ongoing support is likely to be necessary.

Q. What happens in a frenulotomy?

A. The research suggests using scissors is the most effective method of division. It's important to understand that it is a surgical procedure, and comes with risks including infection, bleeding and reattachment, which is why we want to always ensure carrying out the procedure is truly appropriate and necessary.

The baby is given sugar water before and after the procedure. Anaesthetic is not usually given because we want the tongue to move freely after the procedure so the baby can feed immediately and the risk of bleeding is reduced.

The baby is usually swaddled in a towel or blanket, with someone holding the baby's head still. The Frenulotomist will divide the frenulum, which usually takes seconds, some pressure is applied briefly using a sterile gauze, before the baby is returned to the mother to be breastfed.

Some mothers say they notice an immediate difference after the procedure, for others the frenulotomy is only the beginning of the journey to improve breastfeeding.

Q. What about lip tie?

A. There is no evidence that a lip tie affects breastfeeding. According to research, the presence of a frenulum that is visible when you lift the top lip is normal anatomy and is likely to retract as the mouth grows, and teeth emerge.

Q. What is the latest research into tongue tie? i.e. What causes it and benefits v risks of division?

A. In recent years there has been a massive increase in the number of babies undergoing frenulotomies. It's difficult to know if the number of babies affected by ankyloglossia is truly increasing, or if we're quicker and keener to recognise, diagnose and treat the condition.

For some mothers and babies the procedure has a positive impact on breastfeeding, but for others it doesn't. The difficulty we have is identifying the babies who will really benefit from the procedure, and those which need other forms of feeding input and support.

There are various theories about the cause of tongue tie including excess folic acid during gestation contributing to the increasing number of identified tongue ties, but as yet, there is no research to support any theory, and more research is definitely required to further our understanding.

Because of the lack of agreement about which tool to use to identify ankyloglossia (tongue tie) there is potential that any examination is fairly subjective on the part of the practitioner, and there is real risk of both over and under diagnosis and treatment. It is a confusing, and controversial subject.

Q. Who do I see if I suspect my baby has a tongue tie?

A. Ultimately, if you're having any difficulties with feeding your baby it's a good idea to find your local IBCLC; we are specialists in all things infant feeding, and can help with any questions or concerns, as well as complex feeding situations.

If you decide to see a Frenulotomist (someone who divides tongue ties) try and find someone who is also an IBCLC, as they will be able to help with feeding input both before, and after the procedure, as well as the division itself.

Creating a birth/feeding plan that supports breastfeeding

1) Colostrum harvesting from 36 weeks. Frozen in syringes and taken to hospital- labelled with name, date and hospital number.

2) Am I confident in hand expressing? Antenatal practice.

3) How will I cope at night? What do I need to hand? Breast pads, lighting, cushions, spare clothes, drink, snacks, nappy changing equipment.

4) How can I delegate chores? Who can do laundry, cleaning, cooking?

5) What are my feeding goals?

6) If supplementation is needed, I would like to use donor milk before formula.

7) Keep open communication with my partner- how can they support me to reach my feeding goals? Limit visitors, hydrate and nourish me, babywear, change baby's nappy.

8) Who is in my support network?

Facebook infant-feeding groups

IBCLC/Doula

Breastfeeding helpline

Breastfeeding café.

9) How does my birth plan support breast/chest feeding? Immediate skin to skin until baby has had first feed, if c-section have leads on back to allow skin to skin, all baby checks to be done whilst skin to skin, baby to be tucked between me and hospital

gown so we both stay warm, laid-back feeding, ensure all hospital staff are aware of harvested colostrum and where it's stored to avoid formula supplementation.

10) How can visitors help? Cooking, dog walking, laundry, childcare (NOT feeding baby!).

11) Feeding plan to log nappy output and feeds (Means I have something to show community midwives or anyone who suggests unnecessary supplementation).

12) If formula supplementation is suggested, can I seek additional help first? Can I use donor milk? Can I use harvested colostrum? Can I pump/hand express?

Lou's breastfeeding checklist

✓ Nappy output.

✓ Frequency of feeds 8-12 in 24 (length irrelevant!).

✓ Sucks and swallows (bursts of 1:1 followed by 2/3:1).

✓ Weight gain or loss?

✓ Do you have pain?

✓ How is the baby?

✓Positioning and attachment checklist-sustainable/chin leading and nipple up nose when approaching/more areola visible above baby's top lip/no space between you both/chin indented into breast/nose free.

✓ Would Cranial Osteopathy help release some neck and head tension to help baby feed?

Lou's Top Tip: Weigh baby on their front (prone weighing)- they seem to cry less this way... adrenaline levels are lower for baby and parents. Baby also wriggles less so you get a quicker, more accurate measurement and baby doesn't have to spend as long away from her parents. You can also use a t-shirt that smells of you on the scales. Take a photo of the measurement to avoid confusion. Don't forget, babies whose mothers have received fluids in labour can lose more weight.

Chapter 6

Bring a Bottle

What equipment do you need?

1. Bottles! There are many different baby bottles on the market and what suits one baby won't necessarily suit the next. Also, just because you spend more on a bottle that promises to do fancy things, like reduce colic, doesn't necessarily mean your baby will prefer this or that it'll work miracles! Sometimes the cheapest are just as good. Bottles tend to come in two different sizes, holding 4-5oz and 8-10oz. You can buy glass (heavy and can shatter), plastic (ensure its BPA free) and silicone (expensive and harder to find) bottles.

   The amount of formula and the number of feeds in 24 hours suggested on the back of a tin is calculated on baby's age and weight. However, this is just a guide and often, particularly in the first couple of weeks, the tin suggests very large amounts. Every baby is unique and it is much kinder to baby and her tummy if we offer smaller more regular feeds (8-12 feeds in 24 hours). Therefore, buying a smaller sized bottle to begin with is a good choice as it reduces the risk of overfeeding. Then as your baby grows and takes larger, more infrequent feeds you may wish to switch to a larger bottle. The takeaway here is to not obsess over amounts of formula, but to watch your baby, their nappy output, weight gain and general health and feed responsively following baby's cues.

2. Teats come in different sizes with the lower the number on the teat the slower the flow of milk (Size 1 slow, Size 3 fast). If you're solely formula feeding then follow your baby's cues on when to move up a teat size. If they become irritable at the bottle then this may be a sign you need to increase the size. Similarly, if your baby gulps and splutters at the bottle then the teat flow may be too fast. Some babies prefer latex teats, whilst others prefer silicone so it can be a case of trial and error. It is best to stick to a slow flow teat if you're combining breastfeeding with bottle feeding so that baby doesn't get used to a faster flow of milk. There are several other factors to consider if you're combi feeding, such as choosing a short to medium sized teat- this ensures the teat goes deep into the baby's mouth, but not so much they'll gag. Also, the width of the base of the teat needs to be of medium size, so most of the teat is in the baby's mouth and his lips are close to the screw cap- baby has to open his mouth wide this way as with breastfeeding. Teats with a rounded tip are also recommended, as opposed to ones with a slanted end. However, the key message here is PACE THE FEED. There is no strong evidence to

suggest nipple confusion is a thing, it is more a case of the baby getting used to a faster flow of milk from the bottle and this having a negative impact on breastfeeding.

3. Bottle and teat brush to clean your bottles thoroughly before sterilisation.

4. Steriliser- there are a number of sterilisers on the market but generally speaking your options are:

UV steriliser- the UV light kills 99.9% of germs without the use of chemicals.

Cold water steriliser- you will have a bucket with a lid on which you fill with water and a sterilising tablet. The solution will need to be changed every 24 hours. All feeding equipment will need to be fully submerged with no air bubbles for at least 30 minutes and the bucket contains a floating cover to help.

Steam steriliser- the water is heated to boiling point and the steam then kills bacteria. These are placed in the microwave or are electric and plugged in. Care must be taken to ensure the openings of all bottles and teats are facing down into the steriliser.

Sterilising by boiling- you will need to make sure what you're boiling won't melt and be aware that teats deteriorate quicker with this method of sterilisation. You can place all bottle-feeding equipment in a pan of boiling water, fully submerged for at least 10 minutes.

Sterilising bags- same process as a steam steriliser but useful for travel as they're compact and lightweight. These come with tick boxes on the back which you need to mark off after every use as they have a limited life.

5. Formula powder/ready-made formula- You can buy powdered formula which you make up as you need, or ready-made formula which you just need to warm up. Remember to always follow the manufacturers individual guidelines on when used milk needs to be discarded and how to make up a feed. There is no need to move through the stages of formula- Stage 1 for the first year is fine. Also, the brands are all very similar so UNICEF state it doesn't matter which one you choose. From six months your baby can have small amounts of full fat pasteurized cow's milk in their solid food and as a drink from the age of one.

How do you make up a bottle safely?

1. Ensure bottle has been sterilised according to manufacturer's instructions.
2. Boil kettle using 1 litre fresh tap water (not water that has previously been boiled). Bottled water contains too much sodium. Use the boiled water within 30 minutes. This ensures the water remains at least 70°c to kill any bacteria in the formula powder.
3. Ensure the area you are making up the feed on is clean.

4. Wash your hands.

5. Keep the teat and cap in the lid of the steriliser, not on the work surface itself.

6. Pour required amount of water into the sterilised bottle. Get down to the level of the bottle to ensure level of water is correct or the concentration of the milk could be affected.

7. Once water is in the bottle then add correct amount of formula powder, using an upturned knife to level off the powder in the scoop.

8. Using the tongs from inside the steriliser, pick up the edge of the teat and put it onto the top of the bottle, and then screw the ring on top.

9. Place the lid on the bottle and swirl (not shake) until dissolved.

10. Cool the milk down by holding under running water.

11. Check temp of milk on inside of wrist, it should feel warm but not hot.

12. A feed should be made up fresh but if this is not possible then ready-to-use formula should be used.

13. The Department of Health states that if using a vacuum flask of boiled water to make up feeds away from home then the flask should be filled full, securely sealed and used within three hours to ensure it remains >70°c. Experiments have shown that if a flask isn't full the temperature of the water can drop more rapidly.

14. Any infant formula left in the bottle after a feed should be discarded within a specific amount of time as stated by the manufacturer.

> Lou's Top Tip: When washing up used bottles always swill in cold water first before washing in hot soapy water, as hot water bakes the milk onto the bottle!

Paced Bottle Feeding

This is a method of bottle feeding that slows the flow of milk, allowing baby to assess when she's full and ensures the caregiver respects this, creating healthier eating habits for the future. It also avoids a scenario where baby gets used to a fast flow of milk with a shallow latch at the bottle (negatively impacting breastfeeding).

1. Feed baby when they show signs of hunger- rooting, hands in mouth, waving arms etc.
2. Hold baby close in the crook of your arm in an upright position, facing you. We want her to be able to control the pace of the feed and we need to watch closely for signs she needs a break. We can also promote language development by talking to her about what's happening.
3. Softly rub the teat against baby's top lip. If baby opens their mouth then gently insert the teat. (If you're combi feeding then keep the bottle lowered, then once baby has sucked a few times then raise the bottle to a horizontal level so the milk is just covering the hole at

the end of the teat. This mimics a let-down when breastfeeding).

4. Keep the bottle in a HORIZONTAL position (only slightly tipped with milk just covering the hole) to prevent milk from flowing too fast.

5. If baby is gulping then lower the bottle to slow the flow down.

6. Baby should pause to breathe every few sucks. Lower the bottle every time baby takes a pause.

7. Follow baby's cues for when they need a break (frowning, arching their back, widening of the eyes, fist clenching) and gently remove the bottle. Try giving them a wonky wind.

8. Half-way through the feed swap sides to promote muscle development and mimic breastfeeding.

9. As the bottle empties take care to ensure the teat isn't bent (you may need to change the position of the bottle, baby or both to avoid this).

10. Never force baby to finish a feed, follow them.

Lou's Top Tip: To compare the difference between traditional bottle feeding, where baby is lying almost flat to feed, and paced bottle feeding fill a baby bottle with water. Holding it over the sink tip the bottle at a downward 45° angle and watch the water flow. Now move the bottle so it is in a horizontal position and take note of the difference in speed that the milk flows.

This is why we want to pace feed!

Elevated side lying feeding

This is a method of feeding which is very useful for both premature babies and newborns who are struggling to bottle feed. Perhaps they have an oral motor disorder or are struggling with the suck, swallow and breathe mechanism.

The pillow supports the baby so he doesn't need to work at controlling his body, he is lying at a natural position similar to that of breastfeeding, the caregiver can watch clearly for baby's signals and any excess milk can dribble out of the side of baby's mouth reducing the chance of coughing/choking.

IBCLC Stacey Zimmels also states on her website that it is kinder on the baby's tummy; *'This is a great position for babies who have reflux or who are prone to vomiting. If you place the baby on its left side to feed it increases the space from the bottom of its stomach to the oesophagus making it less likely for them to vomit or reflux.'*

It can be used for both formula fed and combi fed babies.

Here's how to do it;

1. Get yourself comfortable on a chair or sofa with a footstool under your feet. Your knees need to be elevated and your thighs at a 45° angle. Place a cushion on your thighs and cover it with a muslin.
2. Place baby on her left side with her head towards your knees, her bottom touching your tummy, her legs and arms out to the side and her ear/shoulder/hips in line.

3. Bring the bottle across so it's horizontal with the floor and rub the teat across baby's top lip. Wait for her to open her mouth to the widest point and draw in the teat herself.
4. Watch baby's cues for when they need a break/wonky wind and take care that as the bottle empties her neck doesn't hyperextend.

Chapter 7

Poo, Poo and more Poo

You are going to become obsessed with poo over the next few months! Checking your baby's nappy output and colour can tell you lots about the health of your baby and how well feeding is going.

First off, how to change a nappy:

Step 1: Get prepared. Lay everything that you're going to need out ready. So, pull some baby wipes out of the pack (or cotton wool, water and a clean flannel if you're using these), open up a nappy sack, and fold open the nappy ready to go on fresh. You might even want to have some spare clothes near in case of an explosion and some cream for sore bottoms.

Step 2: For babies on the move changing on the floor is always safest, but otherwise using a changing table is fine particularly if you've had a caesarean and can't bend down (just don't leave your baby unattended). Lay baby on the mat on their back and undress their bottom half, remembering to remove socks as babies have a habit of putting their feet in their poo!

Step 3: Undo the tabs on either side of the nappy and pull the front down wiping the nappy against the skin as you go to remove initial stool residue. Then tuck the front part of the nappy under baby's bottom so that any remaining poo makes its way onto the dirty nappy rather than the changing mat. You can then lift baby's legs up gently by holding her ankles and start to wipe her bottom, from front to back so as not to spread poo into vagina, with the wipes/cotton wool remembering to clean all the creases. Once the majority of the poo is off you can remove the dirty nappy, roll it up and secure it with the stick tabs before popping it in the bin. Then give baby a final wipe over to ensure they're completely clean. Dry the area with a clean flannel and apply cream if needed. Babies tend to love a nappy-free kick about but just beware they may tinkle on you!

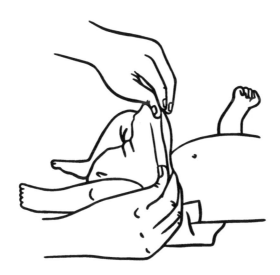

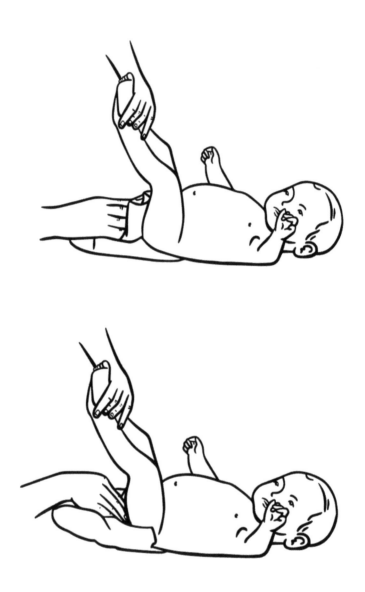

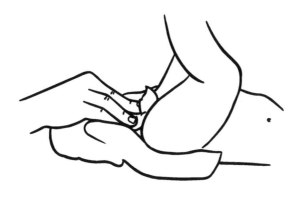

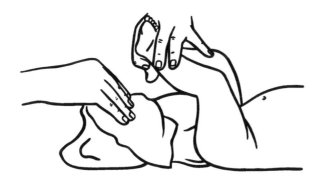

Step 4: Take the unfolded clean nappy, lift baby's legs up again gently holding his ankles and shuffle the back of the nappy underneath up to his waist. Then lift the front part of the nappy up and over the front, ensuring if you have a boy his penis is tucked down, and fasten the tabs over the front to secure. You don't want the nappy to be too tight so ensure you can still fit a finger down the top edge of the nappy. Finally remember to uncurl the edges of the nappy that go between her legs to avoid chafing and to help prevent leakage. Put your baby's clothes back on.

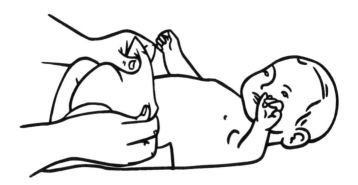

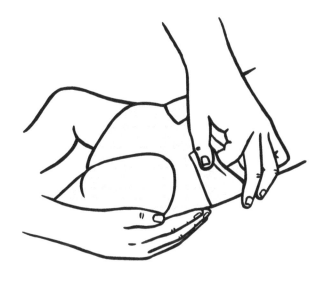

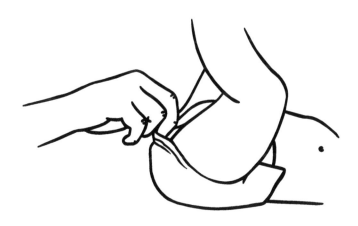

Step 5: Place baby somewhere safe and clear up. Don't forget to wash your hands thoroughly.

Your baby's first poo is called Meconium and it is a bit like the colour and texture of Marmite. Meconium is made up of substances your baby swallowed in the womb such as amniotic fluid, skin cells and mucus. Roughly between days 2-4 the colour of your baby's poo will transition towards a dark green (like Pesto) through to a yellowy brown (like Chicken Korma) as the milk is digested. Formula fed babies have poo the texture of toothpaste which can be yellow-tan and smelly. Breastfeed baby's poo is runnier with a seedy/runny like appearance that smells sweet. Some parents panic if their breastfed baby's poo turns green but as long as this isn't happening consistently and baby seems well in himself then this is normal.

Please see your GP if your baby has blood in their poo. Baby's poo can appear shiny and stringy with mucus when they're teething as mucus in the saliva can be undigested, and similarly if they have a cold due to the excess mucus. However, if this is happening regularly then again it is always wise to get it checked by the GP.

It is also normal for newborn baby girls to have a small period a few days after being born. This is nothing to worry about and is due to a surge in hormones which stimulate your baby's womb to produce a false period.

Urates might also appear in your baby's nappy. Also known as 'brick dust' this is made up of substances from the urine that form and crystalise. It will appear as a dark pink/red stain in baby's nappy. It can be a sign that the baby is dehydrated, as the urine is more concentrated, so if baby continues to pass these beyond the first couple of days then seek medical advice.

To check your baby is having enough wet nappies take a nappy and fill it with 3tbsps water. This will give you an indication of how heavy the nappies should feel when you change them.

Your baby's minimum nappy output should look like this:

Day	Wet	Dirty
1	1	1-2
2	2	2
3	3	2
4	4	2
5	5	2
6 onwards	6	2

Lactation Consultant Philippa Pearson-Glaze who founded the wonderful evidence-based website breastfeeding.support states *'A breastfed baby's pattern of dirty nappies can change around six weeks of age and they may start having fewer dirty nappies or not pooping every single day. Wambach and Spencer explain that the ratio of whey to casein (milk proteins) in breast milk changes slightly around six weeks resulting in slightly thicker more formed stools that may be passed less often although many patterns of stooling are possible.*

Lactation Consultant Robyn Noble says a breastfed baby over six weeks of age will typically have one copious mustard yellow poop per day with a consistency of toothpaste.'

Again, keep an eye on the number of wet nappies and weight gain.

You may also notice your baby cries, goes red, appears to strain or groan when he's pooing or trying to poo. Newborns need time to develop the coordination between brain, muscles and pelvic floor in order to poo. As long as the poo is soft when it arrives, and your baby is otherwise gaining weight and healthy, then this isn't normally a cause for concern. You can always try gently massaging their tummy in a clockwise direction following their line of digestion, placing your baby's feet together (soles touching) and rocking his feet up towards his nose and back again, or rubbing the soles of the feet in a circular motion for relief. If you're worried, always seek help from a medical professional.

Chapter 8

Splash, Splosh, it's Bath Time

Bath time provides a multitude of benefits for your baby. The warm water reminds her of the womb world, language development is promoted as you talk to her and her senses of sight, sound and touch are stimulated.

Don't worry if it takes a few tries before your baby enjoys the experience- this is normal. Keep it short and try again in a couple of days, perhaps taking a bath together next time. Ensure you choose a time when she isn't hungry or tired, and that her cord stump has dropped off first.

It is normal to feel anxious about bathing your newborn. Your newborn is fine with topping and tailing until you feel more confident, which is where you wash their face and bottom using cotton wool and luke-warm boiled water.

How to bath your baby:
1. Ensure room is warm and baby is content. Run a bath (temp 36-38c and depth 8-10cm) NB without bubble bath.
2. You will need a bowl of luke-warm boiled water (can use tap water after 1 month), cotton wool balls, a towel, a fresh nappy and clean clothes.
3. Take off the baby's clothes, leaving her nappy on, and wrap her in a towel. Start with her eyes- wipe from her nose outward (to avoid any spread of infection) over each eye using a new cotton wool ball per wipe. Next clean around her ears, over her nose and around her mouth.

4. Now baby can go in the bath. Use your elbow or a bath thermometer to check the temperature of the bath (it should feel like your body temperature). Then you can take her out of the towel and nappy and place her in the bath.
5. To hold baby safely put one hand under her shoulders and neck, and the other hand supporting her bottom.
6. Wash her body, talking to her all the while, and then her hair last to prevent her getting cold.
7. Be extremely careful when removing her from the bath as she will be slippery.
8. Dry thoroughly in all the nooks and crannies, get her dressed and wrap her in a blanket to keep warm (weather dependent).

NEVER leave your baby unattended in the water.

There is no need to use any soap, at least until the baby is 6 weeks old, as this removes natural oils and dries the skin out.

When filling the bath for a baby always put cold water in first, then top up with hot. Finish off with cold so that if any water drips from the tap onto baby it won't scold them.

Babies only need to be bathed 2-3 times a week.

You may like to take a bath with your baby, a fantastic opportunity for skin to skin but do ensure someone else is there to hand baby to you and take her at the end.

Chapter 9

Sling-a-bye Baby

Slings and carriers are an absolute godsend and I use them daily in my postnatal work. They provide a multitude of benefits to both you and your baby and can be used for years well beyond babyhood! They support baby in adapting to the big wide world and meet his need for security and a strong attachment. Slings help soothe baby-he can hear your heartbeat and smell you which can be very reassuring. Carrying also helps regulate baby's temperature whilst he's next to you and can help baby bring up wind.

Carrying nurtures the parent baby dyad and increases responsive feeding and parenting. By being closer to your baby you are more likely to pick up on his hunger and tiredness cues. Having your baby close keeps levels of Oxytocin (the love hormone) high, which will aid breastfeeding and encourage bonding.

The motion babies experience whilst in the sling helps their vestibular apparatus develop, aiding balance, and when correctly worn they support the development of a healthy spine and hips. Language development is also promoted as you talk to baby whilst you carry him. Another benefit is that the caregiver is hands free which is really helpful when you need to run an errand or look after siblings.

There are a number of things to remember when carrying your baby in a sling or carrier. The baby's hips should be well supported to avoid hip disorders and this is achieved when the legs are in a frog or 'M' shaped position. The fabric of the sling or carrier should run underneath baby's bottom and into the knee pit (so that the knees are lifted and baby's bottom is lower). Once baby is in the sling you can ensure they're at the optimum M shaped position by imagining baby's thighs are glasses of water which you're going to pour away. Hold your baby's thighs and 'pour the water away'. This will cause the hips to tip, raising baby's knees and lowering his bottom. Adjust any loose straps where necessary.

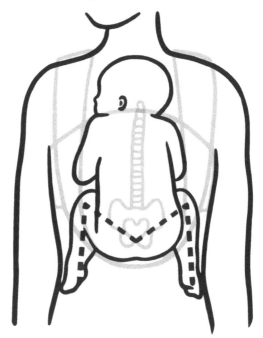

Ring slings can be used from birth and allow baby to adopt the natural curved foetal position and are great for breast and bottle-feeding access. However, care must be taken to ensure baby's airways are clear; two fingers should always fit between their chin and their chest.

Avoid tying material across baby's back as this can cause unnecessary pressure on your baby's spine.

If there is any loose material, the carrier leaves red marks on your baby, is painful for you to use or if a sling that crosses over your back starts to ride up then the sling needs to be readjusted or perhaps isn't the right one for you.

You need to take care to ensure you do not fall asleep with your baby in a sling- their airways need to be regularly checked.

Always follow the TICKS:

Tight enough to hug your baby, otherwise he will slump down into the carrier which can hinder breathing

In view so you're able to always check on them and their face isn't covered with any material

Close enough to kiss. This ensures baby is high up enough on your chest

Keep baby's chin off chest otherwise breathing is restricted. There should be at least a finger's width space under his chin

Supported back. The baby should be in a natural position with his chest and tummy against yours. If when you press gently on his back he moves closer to you or appears to uncurl, then the sling is too loose and the baby is slumped

I can highly recommend finding your local Sling Library (www.ukslinglibraries.wordpress.com) or Sling Consultant so that you can try on some different slings/carriers and see which one suits you best. Many of my clients buy two as one parent prefers one particular carrier compared to another.

I asked Sling Consultant and Doula, Lucy Pedder from Derbyshire for her top tips on choosing a sling for your baby and here's what she had to say:

'The range of slings and carriers available is staggering and can be very overwhelming. It's a huge industry that can sometimes seem to prey on parents' doubt and worry, with fancy, expensive carriers offering a host of safety features and adjustable, removable, addable, upgradable, parts and functions. However, humans have been strapping babies to our torsos with fabric since we lost our body hair and invented textiles tens of thousands of years ago. It doesn't have to be that complicated. Think about how you naturally hold your baby on your chest, with their back gently curved, knees tucked up, head under your chin, maybe little hands balled on your chest or close to their mouth. This is the cosy, close secure position we are wanting to achieve and that your baby will naturally adopt, given the right support. For newborns a stretchy

wrap or a ring sling is ideal. Both take a little bit of practice to get right but once you have understood how they wrap around you and your baby it becomes the easiest thing in the world to pop your sling on in the morning and then your baby can move in and out as and when needed. Ring slings are particularly handy as you can put one on OVER your sleeping or fractious child in your arms, without having to put them down first to sort the sling out. For slightly older or heavier babies, right up to toddlers, woven wraps are hard to beat. The length of a stretchy wrap with the stability of a ring sling, woven wraps can carry a tiny baby on your chest, a nosy eight month old on a hip or a rambunctious 2 year old on your back. There is a misconception that you need a "wrap" or "sling" for indoors and a more structured "carrier" for hikes and shopping trips. This is completely untrue. Any device that holds your baby safely against your body and is comfortable and supportive for both you and your child can be used for 5 mins while you make a sandwich in your kitchen or for several hours while you hike up a mountain. Some parents find the buckles and straps of a carrier more reassuring and easy to understand, others prefer the infinite adjustability of a wrap. Either way, it's possible to turn babywearing into an all-consuming, money-sapping obsession, collecting the latest designs and prints and acquiring a new sling for every season and every age and developmental stage your baby passes through. This is fine if you are something of a collector and this becomes a fun hobby, but it isn't necessary, and your baby won't benefit. As a sling consultant I own a large laundry bag of different slings and carriers to demonstrate to and help my clients with, but as a postnatal doula I carry ONE woven wrap into which I can pop any child I encounter as needed! Whatever your body shape, physical needs and those of your child; babywearing offers massive benefits for the whole family and can be a vital parenting tool. Make use of sling libraries and invest in a consultation with a babywearing expert to find the sling that suits your needs, your baby and your body best. Happy babywearing!'

Chapter 10

Two Peas in a Pod

As a non-identical twin myself, I've always had a real interest and soft spot for multiples and have been lucky enough to work with both twins and triplets.

Did you know? Around 40% of multiples need some extra help in hospital after the birth in the form of the special care baby unit. If only one baby requires care, then the staff should do their utmost to keep the babies together. Your babies will be cared for by specialist nurses who will ensure the babies are kept at the correct temperature, given oxygen if they need support breathing and fed via a feeding tube if necessary. Your multiples will benefit hugely from skin to skin, so ask the nurses to help with tucking them under your top against your skin. The special care baby unit can be quite a noisy place with all the machinery and you may well be feeling overwhelmed and anxious. It is important that lines of communication are kept open and if you have any questions that you ask the staff. The staff should fully prepare you for what to expect when you get home with your babies and if any medication needs to be administered etc. Where possible try not to assign one baby with one carer- it is great for bonding if you swap.

Multiples will love sleeping together and find this very reassuring and soothing, after all this is what they've been used to in the womb. I'm convinced one of the reasons why I like sleeping with lots of duvet over my head is because my sister spent nine months on top of me!! Remember to still practice safe sleep guidelines, such as feet to foot and placing babies to sleep on their backs. It is important to remember they are individuals and that one baby may like being patted to sleep whilst the other baby hates it. Don't forget to check out the sleep environment section of the book as this is still very important.

Slings are going to be invaluable to you just the same way as they are for parents with one baby. Many parents find they prefer to build up their confidence carrying just one baby at a time first before moving on to tandem babywearing. The other baby could be worn by someone else or pushed in the pram. Visiting your local sling library or tracking down your local sling consultant should be a priority. There are a number of slings on the market, some which allow you to carry both one and two babies, others which are specifically designed for multiples. Some people manage to find a way of wearing two individual slings at the same time to carry twins! Baby chairs are also a great purchase as they allow you to put one baby down in a safe place whilst you attend to the other(s).

Don't forget that you might be able to access free support from the childcare department at your local college or Homestart (a network of trained volunteers and expert support that helps families with young children). Looking into this antenatally can take the pressure off. Setting up a rota so that you have someone visiting each day can really help and working out who is going to be in charge of laundry, walking the dog, shopping etc.

Last but not least, you will be a celebrity wherever you go from now on! So, prepare yourself for the inevitable questions; 'Are they identical?' 'Were they IVF?' 'Do multiples run in your family?' 'How do you tell them apart?' and the worst of all 'How on earth do you cope?'.

The lovely Karly Proverbs (Mum of twins, Osteopath, FEDANT Infant Feeding Coach and Mummy MOT Practitioner) very kindly shared with me her top ten tips for expecting twins:

So, you're expecting twins…Congratulations!!! The way you look after your twins will be as individual as you are. Some people have twins and feel calm and totally prepared for them. Some people have older children and are then surprised with the double blessing that twins are. Some, like myself, have been through IVF and have had the joy (and shock) of being told that both embryos are viable and you're pregnant with twins.

I spent a lot of time preparing checklists of how I would cope when I was pregnant. I felt really prepared in some respects but totally ill-prepared in others. I hope these tips will be helpful and will help you to enjoy the early days with your two precious bundles.

1. *Join your local Twins club*

   I was fortunate enough to join the Greenwich and Lewisham Twins Plus Club when I was pregnant and have made some amazing friends who I still see on a regular basis! There is nothing quite like having a cup of tea with a fellow parent of multiples and know they really, really understand how overwhelming it can feel to get out of the house in the early days. They also get how amazing it is to look down at two sleeping babies that are both yours! Twins Clubs often have buying and selling Facebook pages, a fantastic way to save some money.

   If you're not sure where to start, have a look on the Twins Trust website. The Twins Trust has a wealth of information on its website including a comprehensive list of the hospitals that have specialist Twins/Multiples clinics, information on work and financial support, birth preferences, parenting school age twins and twin discounts. They've also got a dedicated Twinline which is free to call where you will get support and advice from fellow parents of multiples. If you can afford to join the Twins Trust it's well worth the annual fee.

2. *Get your house in order before your twins arrive*

   Talk to your partner about household chores and how they will be divided once your multiples arrive. It's difficult looking after one baby, not to mention two or more and it certainly takes more of your time. Getting your finances in order before your babies arrive is a really good idea. This includes thinking about how you pay your bills as well as childcare depending on your work situation(s). It's a sad fact that many of us with multiples never go back to work or do so on a part time basis. It's often cheaper for one parent to stay at home and look after the children because the cost of childcare is more than what one parent earns. It's also worth making sure your wills are up to date, it's macabre but it's important.

Batch cooking and freezing meals means you don't have to think about what to prepare for supper. Can your partner make your lunch before they head off for work? A cup of tea in an insulated flask or mug is also one of the nicest things your partner can make for you. It's a simple thing but it can be a huge help when you're elbow deep in nappies and trying to wash yet another load of baby laundry. Working as a team is essential whether you are having one baby or three so it's important to talk about how you might divide your household chores.

3. Buggy – try before you buy!
Twin buggies are an essential piece of kit for getting around with your two little ones and the one you choose really depends on your lifestyle. If you do have a local twins club it's definitely worth getting in touch with them and pushing the different styles of buggy around. See if you can push their twins in the buggy so you really get an idea of whether that model works for you.

It's also important to measure the width of your front door so you can be confident that you're able to get in and out of the house without having to collapse the buggy. It's worth considering whether you have steps outside your door. If you do, plan how to get out of the house with your buggy and the twins. Alternatively, you might want to keep your buggy in the car in which case make sure you get a buggy that doesn't have air filled tyres or they will deflate on a hot day (I speak from experience!).

4. Sleeping

Having two cot beds for your twins from day one isn't always necessary. I put my twins in the same cot bed until they started rolling over at around four months postpartum. They were positioned feet to foot so that they were at opposite ends of the cot bed in age and tog appropriate sleeping bags.

The Twins Trust has a helpful safer sleeping factsheet. It's free to download and has been produced in conjunction with the Lullaby Trust for keeping twins and triplets safe while sleeping. I slept in the spare room with my twins until they were over six months so I wouldn't disturb my husband during the night feeds.

During the day I let my twins nap in a travel cot downstairs so I could keep a close eye on them. I also set up a changing station downstairs which was particularly helpful after having an emergency c-section. It meant I could pop them in the travel cot and get some chores done or crash on the sofa too. If you live in a house, it's worth having a similar set up in the early days.

5. _Feeding_

If you can, it's worth seeking the advice of an Infant Feeding Coach or IBCLC **before** your twins arrive. I had fantastic care from my specialist twin midwife, attended an online breastfeeding webinar with the Twins Trust and read extensively but really struggled with breastfeeding. If I could go back in time, I would have sought out individual help at the beginning of my third trimester so I was better prepared for feeding my twins.

Feeding twins is always a challenge but speaking to a professional who can provide you with evidence-based advice and guidance will help to minimise the stress associated with feeding not one but two or more small little mouths when you are exhausted and overwhelmed.

6. _Pack your bag from 26 weeks_

Deciding where you will have your baby can be a complex decision, you may have to travel further or you might be close to two hospitals that have twin clinics. It's down to personal choice and it's important to trust your instincts. The Twins Trust website has a list of hospitals which have designated twin clinics so it's a good place to start.

Pregnancies with multiples are considered higher risk than singleton pregnancies so you will have more scans and hospital appointments. Multiples often arrive early so it's certainly worth having your bag packed by week 26 just in case. It feels very early but it does mean there is one less thing to think about. That said, being pregnant *with multiples doesn't mean you cannot have a healthy pregnancy, but it does mean that you will feel pretty exhausted towards the end.*

You might want to see if you can have a tour of NICU even if it's virtual as there is a higher probability of your multiples ending up in NICU. Not all multiples require intensive care but you may feel better prepared if you see it first.

7. *Be organised*
When I asked my fellow twin and triplet parent friends how they managed with their newborns, the most common answer was to try to be as organised as possible. This doesn't mean you shouldn't feed your tiny babies on demand, but it does mean having a bit of a routine. This might be as soon as possible if you choose to bottle feed your babies or once your milk supply is established if you are breastfeeding.

For me, their bedtime routine was the first thing I introduced when they were six weeks old. Every evening I would give them a quick bath. I bathed one at a time, with one in a bouncer sat next to me in the bathroom and the other in their bath seat, and then swapped them round. Then they would have a feed and I'd pop them into their cot, read them a story and kiss and cuddle them to sleep. As the weeks progressed, they seemed to look forward to their bath and even if they were crabby beforehand the bath would change their mood.

Things like buying your grocery shopping online can save so much time. Set up a favourites list and/or a weekly essentials list when you're pregnant so you can streamline the time it takes you to shop.

I was also fortunate enough to be able to afford and have room for a tumble drier. They are certainly expensive to run but in the early weeks it made washing and drying loads and loads of muslins, sleep suits and bedding so much easier. A heated drying rack is a good alternative too. If you can dry things more quickly it means you will hopefully not have to buy as many. That being said, I don't think you can ever have too many muslins when you have multiples!

8. Get some help
Help can come in many forms and will vary depending on your circumstances. Some twin parents have lots of family and friends around them who can help them on a regular basis. Other twin parents need to hire help. Some twin parents have a mixture of both! There is no right or wrong but it's certainly worth considering your options before your twins arrive. Help means different things to different people and what you would like help with before you give birth might change once your babies have arrived. There is no greater gift than someone coming to visit you and bringing a home cooked meal or taking your twins out in the buggy for a quick walk while they nap so you can have a nap or a shower...probably a nap!

If you are in a position to hire help, think about what might work best for you and your family. Doulas, mother's help, night nannies and nannies (part or full time) are all options. It's worth researching what is available locally and speaking to a few people. It goes without saying that you should feel comfortable with anyone who is supporting you. Fellow twin parents are always full of great recommendations too which is yet another reason to join your local twins club.

If people want to get you a baby shower gift perhaps ask them to donate to a fund which will allow you to pay for an extra set of hands.

9. *Look after yourself*
Having a child is hard physically, mentally, and emotionally and there is twice or more of the fun to be had if you are a multiple mother!

According to Twins Trust, postnatal depression is more common in parents of multiples. It's no surprise given the demands that having more than one baby places on you coupled with the lack of sleep. It's estimated that only 1 in 7 mothers of multiples have 6 or more hours of sleep a night in the first year. A list of symptoms is set out on the NHS website and may include a persistent feeling of sadness and low mood; trouble sleeping at night and feeling sleepy during the day; a loss of interest in the world around you; no longer enjoying things that give you pleasure; problems concentrating; feeling agitated, irritated or apathetic; difficulty bonding with your babies;

frightening thoughts or thinking about self-harm or suicide.

If you think you may be suffering from postnatal depression please get help. You can speak to your midwife, GP, friends or family. Alternatively, help is available via Twinline, the Twins Trust freephone helpline.

Carrying twins is physically demanding. My husband used to remind me that Doctor Who only had 2 hearts and I was pumping blood through 3! The weight of the 2 babies and placenta(s) is also significant. Keep yourself fit through pregnancy and take advice about what to do and then make sure you are properly checked over in the months after the children arrive - I recommend a Mummy MOT check-up from a certified practitioner.

10. *Mindset*

Finding out you are having twins/triplets or more elicits different responses in people. When your babies are small you quickly get used to people asking if multiples run in your family, if they're identical, how they were born, how you manage, how they were conceived and even if they're 'natural' (all babies are natural!). You will also be inundated with comments like "double trouble!!"; "you've got your hands full!"; "rather you than me"; "mine are really close in age so they're just like twins!". There isn't enough room for all the things random strangers have told me but you soon learn to laugh about it.

All babies are blessings but having multiples is quite simply amazing. There will be times when you will look back and wonder how you managed, but you will!

I asked a group of parents on an online multiples group what their recommendations would be for expectant parents of multiples and these were their responses:

'We were super lucky in that we got offered a lot of hand me down clothes- everyone kept saying we'll need loads as we have two babies. But actually we got away with much less clothing than you would expect so I wish I didn't panic gather as much as I did, as I just had to find new homes for it all after. It was a lot of unnecessary organising and sorting that I didn't need.'

'Get a sling!'

'Buy as many muslin cloths as you can!'

'Batch cook as much as you can before they're born. If people are visiting, make it a rule they bring a dish!'

'Ask for vouchers for new baby gifts if you can. You will be inundated with cuddly toys, blankets and clothes when the babies arrive but may need something unforeseen and pricey like a breast pump.'

'Ask someone else to feed you!'

'Put a note on the door with visiting times and state 'Make your own tea and one for me too please!'

'Don't forget to look after yourself too. Keep plenty of water and snacks near.'

'Collect as much colostrum as you can antenatally.'

'Purchase a twin feeding cushion that is the right height and fit for you. I went through three before I found the right one.'

'Be kind to yourself. Having more than one baby is hard. It is ok to just focus on surviving each hour, day etc!'

Lactation Consultant Kathryn Stagg is a mother of twins herself and specialises in supporting families with multiples. I was very fortunate to hold a question and answer session with her:

Q. How do you breastfeed twins?

A. You can breastfeed twins singly, or you can breastfeed them together, one on each breast, this is called tandem feeding. Many twin mums will do a combination of this. There are pros and cons to tandem feeding. Pros are that it takes half the time to feed both babies, and if they are both hungry or unsettled at the same time, you can soothe both of them together without having the stress of one feeding and one crying. Cons are it can be a little more tricky to get a good latch in the early days, and it can be quite overwhelming.

Q. Will I be able to produce enough milk for both babies?

A. Milk production works on a demand and supply basis. The more milk you remove, the more you make. So with two babies stimulating the breast instead of one, you should be able to make enough milk for both. The key is frequent and efficient feeds, so making sure they are feeding enough if they are sleepy and making sure they have a good latch. If babies are early, sometimes we need to add some pumping in to begin with, as they can be a bit inefficient at the breast.

Q. Should I give my babies top ups of formula?

A. The answer is only if they need it and you can't use your own milk. A full feeding assessment should be offered and a feeding plan made in response to how your babies are latching and feeding. Unfortunately, with health care as it is at the moment, they often do not have time to do this and will give generic volumes with no plan to protect milk production. If you are finding that you are being told to top up, but not given any actual breastfeeding support, this can be a good time to seek out a Lactation Consultant or Breastfeeding Counsellor.

Q. How do I pace bottle feed twins?

A. To properly pace bottle feed, you really do have to do it one at a time. So either two parents, or one parent and a helper taking a baby each. You could have their feed times staggered so you can bottle feed singly. All bottle fed twin parents find ways to tandem bottle feed when they need, but it is much more difficult to pace the feeds properly.

Q. Should my babies sleep together?

A. Research shows that twins often settle more easily if they share a sleep space. They have been in the womb together for many months after all! There is also some evidence that they will become more in sync with night waking etc which can be useful if trying to tandem feed so you get the feed over more quickly. A large bedside cot or DIY bedside cot (you can take the side off a standard cot and push it up to the bed to make a large bedside cot) helps you have easy access to the babies to feed and settle them.

Q. Should I buy two of everything?

A. No, you don't need two of everything. One cot is adequate to begin with, for example. You will obviously need more clothes, two car seats, one steriliser if you use bottles, twice as many nappies (looking at reusable can ease the guilt around filling landfill!) but you only need one pram. You can get away with one stretchy wrap and tandem carry if you need to when they're little. Don't forget there is a healthy preowned market too, and you can often get your money back after if you sell an item on again. So much better for the environment than buying everything new.

Q. How will I get any sleep?

A. This is actually the most challenging thing about having twins. You have two different babies, with two different personalities, not necessarily with the same sleep needs! As I said above, twin parents will often wake the second baby and tandem feed at night. However, some prefer to single feed so they can lie down and feed more easily, so it's not always the answer. The main thing is to try to get as much help as you can with everything. Having twins is an extreme parenting situation, so call in all the favours, don't be afraid to ask or to explain what you need.

Q. How do you wind two babies by yourself?

A. If you're tandem feeding using a feeding cushion, you can sit them on the edge, leaning into your shoulder and wind them that way. They don't always need winding at the same time so you will often find twin mums winding one whilst continuing to feed the other. You get very good at juggling babies! However, breastfed babies tend to need less winding so just putting them up on your shoulder often does the trick.

If you're breastfeeding twins there are a number of feeding positions you can try. A double breastfeeding pillow can be really useful but they don't suit all body shapes so you may need to try out a few before you find one that suits. They usually come with a small cushion for you to support your back and the feeding pillow will slope slightly towards you to stop the babies rolling. To start with, have both babies nearby and pick up the first baby and allow him to attach to the breast in the rugby ball position. Once he is latched you should be able to pick up the second baby and position him to feed at the other breast, again in the rugby ball hold:

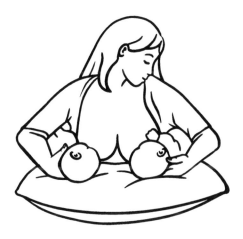

If a feeding pillow isn't for you, you can feed both babies in the biological nurturing/laid back feeding position or position the first baby in the cross cradle hold and the second baby in the rugby ball hold (the baby in the rugby ball hold rests on the baby in the cross cradle hold!). You will need someone to wedge cushions around you for extra support once the babies are attached and feeding:

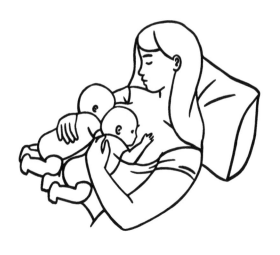

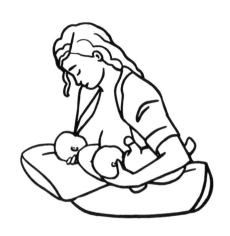

At night you may wish to practise side lying feeding, where one baby feeds lying on his side at one breast and the second baby lies in the rugby ball hold or biological nurturing position across your side feeding from the other breast:

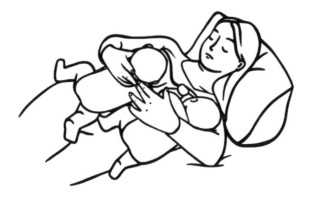

Tandem feeding might help a weaker baby get more milk as it stimulates a let-down. Alternatively, if you're expressing do this whilst the weaker baby feeds.

There are plenty of videos and pictures online at www.breastfeedingtwinsandtriplets.co.uk.

Chapter 11

Ages and Stages

Let's take a look at what your baby's development will look like in the first six months. It is so easy to compare your baby to others because you care so deeply and you just want the best for them. Social media has definitely not helped us with feelings of guilt, anxiety and pressure. However, please remember children all develop at different rates and are all unique. Temperament can also play a part- for example, a baby who is desperate to grasp that toy in the distance is more likely to roll than a baby who is happy to lay on the mat and watch the world go by (as long as they have a full tummy and lots of cuddles too!). If you are at all concerned about anything then always seek help from a healthcare professional.

Newborn

Babies are born with primitive reflexes that occur in response to a stimulus as mentioned earlier. These are replaced by voluntary responses around 3 months of age. As well as the rooting, sucking and swallowing reflexes there are others too. The grasp reflex- baby closes his hand in response to something on the palm of the hand. The stepping reflex- baby makes stepping movements when held up and on a flat surface. The asymmetric tonic neck reflex- if baby's head is turned to the left, the left arm and leg will extend, and the right arm and leg will bend, and vice versa. Moro reflex- triggered by sudden movement, loud noises or abrupt loss of contact with the caregiver; they will fling out their arms with their hands open before bringing them back over their chest as though they're cuddling themselves.

Babies have a preference for people over objects! In Lynne Murray's book 'The Social Baby' she talks more about this; *'Within minutes of birth, the baby can show her preference for contact with people, rather than objects. For example, the baby will turn her head to the sound of someone's voice, when another sound, even if of the same pitch and intensity, will not attract her attention. The baby has already heard voices before she was born, so this response is partly based on her previous experience. But the baby is also attracted to faces, something she has certainly not come across before! Given a choice between looking at a face-shaped pattern, and one with the arrangement of eyes, nose and mouth scrambled up, the newborn baby will spend longer looking at the face.'* And another sign that shows your baby is ready to connect socially is his ability to copy your expression. Try sticking your tongue out or opening your mouth wide whilst looking at your newborn and see if he copies you!

Babies use their senses right from the word go. There have even been experiments done where babies have been placed in a cot and a fan is placed either side. One blows the scent of baby's caregiver and the other another scent.

The babies have been found to turn towards the scent of their caregiver!

<u>1 month+</u>

Your baby will now begin to open his hands from time to time and bring his fists to his mouth. He will make jerky and uncontrolled limb movements and his head will still need to be supported. Your baby will be mesmerised by primary colours lights and sounds. When held in the crook of your arm your baby will stare at you and by around six weeks you should notice his first smile! He may also coo when he sees you and follow objects as you move them; known as tracking, which helps with vision, hand eye coordination and the ability to take on more information.

<u>3 months+</u>

Your baby will now begin to hold her head up for periods during tummy time and you may notice her leaning her head forward in the car seat showing off her new skills! She will begin rolling from her tummy onto her back and gradually gain more control over her hands and arms; holding a rattle for a short time that you'd placed in her hand, and batting and grabbing the toy that takes her interest. Her eyes can now focus on the same point and she will begin to follow you as you walk around the room as her eyesight develops further. You can have lots of fun taking it in turns to talk now too as your baby responds with squeals and gurgles of delight! Between about 3-6 months your baby's Moro reflex will merge into the mature startle reflex, which is there for life and allows baby to better manage their involuntary jump/startle, or perhaps even ignore it.

<u>6 months</u>

By now your baby will be rolling from their back onto their tummy and starting to sit unaided. Most toys find their way to your baby's mouth and they have much better control over their hands enabling them to explore the toys they hold and pass them from one hand to the other. They will be able to hold their head and chest up confidently during tummy time, supporting themselves with their hands and arms. When lying on their back they will love to explore their feet before kicking vigorously! Moving forward they will be able to poke objects with their index finger and lift their arms up as a signal that they want you. Babies of this age love to babble spontaneously, first with monosyllables like 'ga-ga' and then double syllables such as 'goo-ga'.

The most wonderful gift you can give your baby in the first few months at playtime is your tender loving touch and communication. Talk to your baby, maybe read them a book or sing to promote their language development, no matter how silly you sound or feel.

The older they get babies love it when you lose your inhibitions and make them giggle too! Children learn through play- they learn new skills, problem solve and make sense of their world through open-ended experiences which help to develop the brain.

Sensory play has huge benefits for babies. Jean Piaget, a Swiss psychologist, studied cognitive development in babies and young children and found they learn a huge amount about their world by touching, watching, listening and moving. Putting these experiences in place and allowing babies to repeat them over and over lays the foundations for learning as the child grows. These sensory experiences should take place in a loving and safe environment.

We know that newborns are born with blurry vision and can only see about 30cm in front of them- funny that this is the distance of your face when you hold them in the crook of your arm! Placing toys at this distance helps them engage. Anna Franklin, head of the baby lab at the University of Sussex states *'It is a myth that babies see in black and white.'* Studies have found that newborns can see large, intense patches of red on a grey background. *'The early stages of learning to see colour and basic forms happen relatively quickly'* says Alex Wade, professor of psychology at the University of York and an expert in visual processes. Babies only perceive depth when they're several months old and an article in The Guardian written by Nicola Davis in 2017 stated that *'By the age of six months, babies have more or less adult levels of visual acuity.'* The research into what babies can truly see is ongoing!

Some great play ideas for the first few months include:

Primary coloured, bold picture cards.

Tummy time (this helps build neck and shoulder muscles to strengthen head control in preparation for sitting up, crawling and walking).

A mirror (babies love studying faces so what could be better than looking at his own reflection in the mirror?!).

Coloured scarves (talk to them about how it feels, the colour, play peekaboo, run the material over their skin).

Sensory bottles (you can make these at home, fill with lentils/rice/pasta/shells/water, glitter and pompoms).

Water mat (baby can do tummy time on this inflatable mat whilst looking at the patterns and watching the floating toys inside).

Foil blanket (this appeals to the senses as it is shiny and crinkly).

Rattles/Shakers (encourage baby to hold the shaker, talk to him about the noise it makes and sing some songs).

Feathers (tickle baby's arms, hands, tummy, legs, feet and head with the feather and allow him to experience these gentle sensations).

Nursery rhyme CD (can be useful if you need reminding of some of the classics or would like to learn some new songs!).

Brightly coloured touch and feel books (fantastic for baby's sensory exploration but also language development as you talk to him about what's inside).

Playgym (a soft padded mat with toys that hang down over baby such as mirrors, squeaky, musical and crinkly toys).

Ribbon and bells ring (you can talk about the different coloured ribbons and tickle baby with them. Baby can hold onto the ring and as he moves it the bells will ring).

Flashing ball/LED mini spinner (babies are mesmerised by the flashing lights. Some LED spinners gently vibrate too. To be used in short bursts as these can be very stimulating).

Hand/Foot rattles (helps baby recognise their hands and feet and that they have control over them).

Treasure basket (full of natural objects that baby can explore safely with all their senses).

Stacking cups/Shape sorter (teaching baby cause and effect, problem solving and promotes hand eye coordination. Great when baby is sitting up).

Have a look online if there is a parents Facebook group local to you that lists the baby stay and play groups in your area. These are a great way for you to meet other parents and for your baby to have exposure to other toys. Your local Children's Centre should run a weekly timetable of activities for you to go to, usually free of charge, and I would highly recommend checking out the following classes:

Baby massage- offers interaction as you bond and talk to your baby, stimulates and aids the nervous/digestive/circulatory/immune/lympathic/respirat ory/vestibular systems, relief from digestive issues and muscle tension and relaxation.

Swimming- strengthens muscles, stimulates the vestibular apparatus which aids balance, language development promoted as you talk to baby, can relax baby, aids bonding.

Music- UNICEF states *'Music makes a big difference to the baby brain. One study from the Institute of Learning and Brain Sciences detected that after babies listen to music, their auditory and prefrontal cortexes look different. These are the regions of the brain in charge of processing both music and speech. Not only that: when young children interact with others, the positive effects of listening to music have been seen to extend personality traits, like being helpful and cooperative.'*

Signing – www.singandsign.co.uk states the benefits include:
> *- helping to understand your baby's needs, thoughts and ideas.*
> *- reducing frustration (for baby and parent!).*
> *- enhancing early vocabulary and understanding.*
> *- encouraging the development of speech.*
> *- enriching your baby's relationships.*

- building confidence and self-esteem.
-stimulating your baby's intellectual and emotional development.

Chapter 12

Food, Glorious Food!

Welcome to this chapter on the introduction of solid/complimentary foods. Note: I don't call it weaning as this often leads people to think you need to wean OFF milk, when actually milk is still a baby's main source of nutrition in the first year. It is the common term though so I will continue to use it throughout this chapter.

When?

The World Health Organisation strongly recommends exclusive breastfeeding for the first six months of life. It states that from six months, other foods should complement breastfeeding for up to two years or more.

Weaning before this stage is not advised as your baby isn't able to process foods properly due to her immature digestive systems and kidneys. However, from six months your baby's iron levels begin to drop so waiting too long can also have an adverse effect.

The process of weaning is not to wean off milk, but rather to introduce the exploration of new tastes and textures during family mealtimes, alongside your baby's usual feeding pattern, and to enhance key skills such as chewing and speech development.

Many people think that a baby's fascination with watching you eat is a sign he is ready for solids, or that sudden waking during the night is another sign. Babies are very interested in the world around them so watching you eat is just another part of that, not a sign he is ready for solids. They also wake frequently during the night for many reasons- teething/illness/developmental change. Again, not a sign to start offering the big stuff!

If your baby pushes food out with their tongue (known as the tongue thrust reflex) this is a sign he is not yet ready for solids.

Being able to sit up and coordinate their eyes, hands and mouth so they can pick up objects are signs of readiness. This may be past 6 months of age- be led by your baby. More here:

https://www.unicef.org/parenting/food-nutrition/feeding-your-baby-when-to-start-solid-foods

Baby led or Purees?

Baby led weaning allows your baby to feed himself using his hands, giving him complete autonomy regarding how much and how quickly he eats. Generally, parents who follow baby led weaning offer their baby whatever the rest of the family are eating at each meal (avoiding/taking out certain foods baby cannot have of course).

If you choose to go down the puree route you can still give baby this autonomy by following his cues about when he's hungry and never forcing food into his mouth. It is important that your baby doesn't stay on pureed food for too long, progressing to mashed/lumpy foods and finger foods that help with chewing and swallowing skills.

You can combine the two methods offering a mixture of purees and hand-held foods from the get-go too.

Please note: gagging and choking are two different things. A baby has a much stronger gag reflex (to protect them from choking) than an adult so it is normal for them to gag on food whilst they get used to it.

Milk

Breastmilk/Formula is the most important food in your baby's diet for the first year, providing him with most of the calories he needs.

A breastfed baby should continue to be fed on demand. La Leche League states *'Nurse your baby before offering other foods. Your milk remains the single most important food in your baby's diet until his first birthday. Additionally, he is more likely to show interest in new foods if he is not ravenously hungry. At this age, other foods are more for experimentation, play and fun.'*

The Public Health England Start4Life programme suggests that a formula fed baby will have on average around 600ml per day at 7-9 months of age, reducing to around 400ml at 10-12 months, but this is just a guide. Always follow your baby.

Foods to avoid

High levels of salt- dangerous for babies as it can overload their system/cause kidney failure.
Honey- risk of Botulism.

Swordfish/Marlin- high levels of Mercury.

Whole grapes/Cherry tomatoes/Popcorn/Whole nuts/Raw carrot/Hard apple/Celery sticks/Large amounts of peanut butter or anything that could break off in large chunks- choking hazard.

NEVER leave your baby alone with food.

Mineral water- high levels of minerals.

Fenugreek- closely related to peanuts.

Celery/Lupin Flour/Mustard- can cause allergies.

Sugar and artificial sweeteners.

Allergies

Nowadays there is no need to wait several days between introducing new foods and it is not thought that waiting until a child is older will prevent food allergies. However, if there is a family history of allergy or your baby has previously displayed sensitivities to a particular food then medical advice must be sought.

Symptoms of an allergy can include sneezing, pain or tenderness around the face, coughing, wheezing, breathlessness, itchy skin, a raised rash, diarrhoea, sickness, swollen lips/eyes/throat. If these symptoms present themselves then it is best to seek medical attention.

Getting started

- The five things I recommend regardless of how you introduce solids are:
  3 washable aprons with sleeves (one on, one in the wash and one spare). You could also purchase a silicone bib that comes with a pouch for catching dropped food.
  A steamer (far better than boiling vegetables as it keeps more of the nutrients in).
  A highchair with a tray.
  Lots of small Tupperware for freezing leftovers and a marker pen for labelling the contents.
  Free flowing sippy cup or a Doidy cup (this is a slanted, open cup that some babies find easier).
- If you decide to go down the puree route you will need:
  A couple of suction bowls.
  Silicone spoons with chunky handles.
  A mini food processor if you're making purees. I find these are better than hand blenders as you have more control over consistency.
  Ice cube trays.
  Freezer bags.

- Follow your baby's cues. Your baby does not need 3 meals a day to begin with- you can gradually move towards this from about 7 months. Babies have small stomachs so just a few teaspoons/pieces of food will be fine.
- Remember milk is your baby's main source of nutrition so follow his cues for feeds (these may vary depending on his appetite).
- Your baby is more likely to try new foods when he isn't tired or hungry. So, choose a time of day when he is calm and try offering some milk first, so he isn't ravenous.
- A Vitamin D supplement is advised by the NHS.
- He may not take much to begin with but don't worry.
- It can take a baby up to 10 tries before he decides whether he likes something or not!
- You can try lightly cooked/steamed soft vegetables or fruit as well as cooked meat or toast if you're baby led weaning. Keep food large enough for your baby to hold in his fist, with enough poking through for him to chew.
- Freeze purees in a covered ice cube tray, then once frozen pop each cube into a labelled freezer bag and place back in the freezer. Now your ice cube tray is ready to be filled with the next puree!
- Vitamin C is best offered alongside Iron as it helps with its absorption.
- Any leftover milk feed can be used in cooking/added to cereal.

- There is no need to move onto any other stage of milk other than Stage 1. The others are a marketing con!
- From 12 months- 350-400ml dairy (inclusive of whole cow's milk as a drink and any other dairy products). You may choose to offer these alongside breastmilk but don't worry if your toddler has enough from breastfeeding and isn't interested.
- If you wish you can introduce a mid-morning and a mid-afternoon snack from 12 months, but these aren't necessary before this age.
- You can offer tap water in a sippy cup from 6 months (ensure it's free flow as this enables baby to practise sipping, working the muscles used for talking).
- Semi skimmed milk can be given from 2 years old.
- You may wish to attend a first aid course to prepare you for potential incidents of choking.

Ref: NHS
La Leche League
Feeding your baby, Fiona Wilcock
SR Nutrition

Books clients have found useful

- Baby led weaning: Helping your baby to love good food, Gill Rapley & Tracey Murkett.
- What Mummy makes, Rebecca Wilson.

- Feeding your baby day by day, Fiona Wilcock.
- Joe Wicks, Wean in 15.
- River Cottage Baby and Toddler Cookbook, Nikki Duffy.

Chapter 13

Up, Up and Away!

I have travelled the world with families and have compiled a pack list along with some tips that I hope you find useful.

Toiletries

Sponge
Body Wash
Hairbrush
Massage oil/baby lotion
Nail Clippers
Wipes
Nappies
Nappy sacks
Plastic bags/Ziploc bags to prevent spillages in car/on airplane
Nurofen
Calpol
Vitamin D drops
Medicine spoons
Calpol plug in and refills in case baby catches a cold
Thermometer
Teething granules/gel
Sudocrem
Baby bath
Bath thermometer
Breast pump and pads

Travel changing mat
Antibacterial hand gel
Tissues
Swim nappies
Medication e.g. Eczema cream

Clothing

Pyjamas
Vests
Clothes- cool and warm, x2 per day (x3 if no washing facilities)
Socks
Coats
Gloves
Hats- woolly/sunhat
Spare clothes for the nappy changing bag
All-in-one UV protection swimsuit

Extras

Pram
Mosquito net for pram
Parasol for pram
Fan for pram
Insect repellent spray
After bite
Sling
Bibs
Bottles and teats

Sterilising bags

Formula powder/Ready to use formula/Expressed milk

Travel cot

Gro Blind/Bin liners for window in case curtains thin

Blankets

Cot sheets (baby will prefer yours from home that smell familiar)

Sleeping bags

Towels- plus small hand towel for journey in case of spillages/for a freshen up. Dock and Bay sell fantastic towels that dry three times faster than a standard cotton towel

Toys and books

Muslins

Car seat

Adapters *check voltage at destination is strong enough to run equipment you're taking!*

Camera

Baby monitor

First aid kit

Night light/White noise machine

Baby's red book

Passports

Tickets

Pen and paper- for reminders/worries/shopping lists

Lou's Top Tips:

- Check immunisations are up to date for trip.
- Feed during take-off and landing to help reduce discomfort in ears as air pressure changes (landing tends to be more uncomfortable).
- Find out where the local hospital is at your destination.
- Pack essentials in hand luggage in case suitcase gets lost.
- Consider purchasing some packing cubes-these are fabric containers with zips that allow you to keep vests/babygros/outfits/socks separate and organised.
- Keep babies under six months in the shade at all times. The website skincancer.org states '*In their first few months, babies are much more sensitive to sun exposure than adults and older children. Their skin contains little melanin, the pigment that gives colour to skin, hair and eyes and provides some sun protection...*

> *... You may be tempted to reach for the sunscreen, but The Skin Cancer Foundation recommends waiting until the baby is 6 months old before introducing sunscreen. The best ways to keep infants sun safe are with shade and clothing.'* When applying suncream to older babies and children use a make-up brush to apply it to their face- much easier!

What should I pack in my nappy changing bag?

Spare outfits x2 in a Ziploc bag (this ensures spare clothes stay clean but also provides a bag for soiled clothing)
Muslins x2
Nappy changing mat
Baby blanket
Nappies
Wipes
Nappy sacks
Hand sanitiser
Feeding equipment e.g. sterilised bottles, flask of boiling water, formula powder, breast pads, nipple shields, feeding apron
Spare change (nothing worse than arriving late to an appointment and finding you need change to park the car!)
A healthy snack and drink for you
Spare top/outfit for you in case of emergency
Basic baby first aid kit

Notepad and pen (things always spring to mind when you're out and about so being able to write them down helps alleviate stress)

Toiletry bag containing tissues, lipsalve, sanitary towels, paracetamol, hand cream

Chapter 14

You, Me and Us

Becoming a parent is an overwhelming responsibility- it is a metamorphosis. The changes play out in many different ways. These start in pregnancy. Our bodies change, we begin to imagine what baby will look like, how you'll take care of him/her and how you'll parent. Well-meaning friends and relatives begin to fill your head with stories of labour and sleepless nights. Some parents attend every class going, others are happy to go with the flow and learn 'on the job'. There are challenges- perhaps physically we struggle with pregnancy, the way our bodies are changing and the pressure felt to snap back afterwards. Letting go of our old life and adjusting to the new- how different will it feel? What will happen with work? Having to master breastfeeding and lack of sleep. Financial worries. Do we have family and friends to support us? Local groups to attend?

Physically our brain is changing too- Dr Craig Kinsley states *'New research indicates the dramatic hormonal fluctuations that occur during pregnancy, birth and lactation may remodel the female brain, increasing the size of neurons in some regions and producing structural changes in others.'*

After birth some parents feel an instant connection/euphoria and have a blissful babymoon period. For others it is a more gradual process of adjustment and connection.

'Love is a flower and some flowers open immediately, others take time to blossom.' Maddie McMahon, Owner of Developing Doulas.

There are certainly a wide range of emotions to experience. The support of others is so important at this time.

I asked the very knowledgeable and experienced Hannah Ewin, Midwife, Mother of three and owner of Birth Boutique in Warwickshire some questions about what to expect immediately after the birth of your baby.

Q. How might you feel after birth?

A. Whichever way your baby has decided to make an appearance there is one common feeling for every new mum or birthing person immediately after birth... tiredness. If you laboured, there will be muscle aches that you didn't even realise would hurt after birth. Your neck, shoulders and arms can feel incredibly tired if you've used them to hold onto things during contractions, thighs can ache from being in squatting positions and you are simply exhausted from the incredible hard work that your body has just done. Even if your baby has been born by caesarean section (whether planned or not) your body has gone through major surgery, and it needs time to regain energy. If it was a planned caesarean, you may have struggled with sleep the night before surgery simply from the normal anxieties of the day ahead.

You may also experience incredible hunger after a natural birth, particularly if you didn't eat much or vomited during labour. When I say that you feel hungry, for me I think it was the hungriest I have ever felt in my life. I ate and ate for a few hours after birth- I would have even given the hospital meals a Michelin star (they do say that hunger is the best chef!). On average you can burn up to 8000 calories giving birth and if you're breastfeeding on top of that there is a lot of catching up to do. However, as a complete contradiction you may find that you have little appetite after birth. It will come back but listen to your body and only do what feels right. The important thing is that you keep yourself hydrated after birth. If you have had a caesarean section, you will be offered water to sip first and then food will be introduced after a couple of hours. Appetite in the first few weeks can fluctuate but you may notice that you feel very hungry if you are breastfeeding and your baby is having a busy cluster feeding afternoon.

Emotionally, mood can vary massively after birth, and this is not often talked about. You may be feeling euphoric, excited and thrilled to have your baby here or you may be feeling exhausted and relieved that it's over. If your birth didn't go the way you'd hoped, you may even be feeling disappointed and saddened. You may have the overwhelming and immediate love for your baby, or you may feel indifferent, particularly if it was a difficult birth. If you do feel like this, please know that this can be a completely normal feeling and that sometimes it takes time for the love and connection with your baby to grow. If you do feel like this, I would also talk this through with your midwife or health visitor as it may be something that they need to support you closely with.

Baby blues is a common emotional feeling that occurs generally around day three and often ties in with breast milk coming in. You may feel emotional and triggered by the slightest thing, low, sensitive and very tearful. It is due to a crazy cocktail of hormones travelling around your body. You may not want to go out, have visitors round, cry for no reason or for what you think of as a ridiculous reason. I sobbed in the kitchen after I had my first little girl because I saw her scan on our fridge of just her feet. I cried because they were so perfect and tiny. I didn't just cry; it was full blown ugly crying and my husband came rushing in thinking that something terrible had just happened. Let's just say he had a bit of eye rolling relief to see me standing there with the scan in my hand. All jokes aside, the difference between baby blues and postnatal depression is it goes away after a couple of weeks. If you are still experiencing heightened emotional responses, feelings of extreme anxiety, difficulties in falling asleep, intrusive thoughts and not wanting to go out or have people over then you must either talk to your midwife, your health visitor or your GP.

The amount of blood loss after birth and in the first 24 hours often surprises people. It is normal to lose up to 500mls of blood immediately at birth. Maternity pads will need to be changed every couple of hours and you may pass some clots (a normal size clot would be one that is no bigger than a 50p). If you are changing a saturated pad hourly or are suddenly getting large gushes of blood that runs down your legs this is not normal, and you should contact your midwife straight away. Your blood loss will be bright red to begin with and then change to a pinker colour and then brown (just like when you come to the end of a period). You may find you have a few hours where it starts to increase again and then settle if you are breastfeeding your baby very frequently or if you have been quite active. It is also important to note that if you have a caesarean section you will still bleed the same amount after birth. You can bleed after birth for up to 6 weeks. If it stops after 6 weeks and then starts again a few weeks later that is your period returning. It's been a long time since we last saw one of those!

If you have required stitches, you will often be offered (if appropriate) a strong anti-inflammatory that is inserted into your bottom. How lovely! In all seriousness, it's fantastic at taking away discomfort down there and it has a much longer therapeutic effect than taking an oral dose so it's probably worth the awkwardness of a finger up the bum! Stitches need to be kept clean and dry. They are dissolvable and will dissolve over a couple of weeks. Baths can cause them to dissolve too quickly so try to avoid sitting in baths for long periods of time (a quick wash is fine). Change sanitary towels frequently to ensure the area stays clean, and once your blood loss has settled a bit try and lie down a couple of times a day without anything on down there to let the area air. It's also good to have a quick wash every time you open your bowels to minimise the chance of an infection. Signs of infection include a yellow oozing from the site, an offensive smell, extreme tenderness, and redness. It's always good to get your midwife to check your stitches each time you see her postnatally. If she has a concern, she may swab the area to screen for an infection or refer you to the GP or back to the hospital if she has any further concerns.

My top tips for soothing stitches are

- *Pop some sanitary towels in the freezer to act as a cool compress. Alternatively, fill some condoms (didn't think you'd be reaching for those so soon!) with water, pop in the freezer and wrap in kitchen roll to apply a cool compress to the area.*
- *Take regular pain relief if needed.*
- *Get a personalised essential oil blend to help offer pain relief and reduce swelling and tenderness.*
- *Avoid sitting on hard chairs. Furthermore, avoid sitting on rubber rings too! This was old school advice and an older family member may suggest this. It actually makes things worse because you are now causing all the pressure to be focused in a centralised area.*
- *Dry the area with a hair dryer if you can't tolerate patting dry with a towel.*
- *If you have any concerns, please get your stitches checked. You may feel embarrassed to have a check when you don't feel 'presentable' shall we*

say. However, your midwife is very used to checking stiches after birth and I'm sure you will feel much happier knowing that all is well.

Your first wee after birth will often be measured to ensure that you are passing a normal amount. The bladder can sometimes become lazy after birth and retain urine. Therefore, by measuring the amount passed we know all is well. Weeing after birth can be quite 'stingy', particularly if you have a graze or have had stitches. You can minimise the amount of stinging by pouring warm water down over your vulval area as you wee to help dilute the urine and make it less concentrated. Alternatively, having a wee in the shower or a shallow bath also helps. When it comes to the first poo after birth, you may not open your bowels for a couple of days and this is perfectly normal, particularly if you opened them during the birth. Ensure you have a good amount of fibre in your diet, are drinking plenty of water and if the thought of pooing with stitches there feels terrifying then put some tissue in your hand and hold your perineum as you go. I can reassure you that you will not burst your stitches but by holding the area you feel there is some support there. If you have had a caesarean then you will most likely be going home with some laxatives to prevent constipation.

Other common symptoms after birth include:

-Cracked or painful nipples: seek support from a Lactation Consultant, Breastfeeding Counsellor or Peer Supporter.
-Excess sweating: due to the drop in Oestrogen. Wearing cotton clothing, increasing fluid intake, avoiding spicy food and limiting caffeine may help.
-Insomnia: try limiting screen time, reducing caffeine, going for a short walk or practising meditation.
If you feel you may be suffering from PTSD then you may like to seek the help of a Cognitive Behavioural Therapist or a Postnatal Doula who will sit with you and allow you to debrief your birth.
Do not hesitate to seek medical attention if you're worried.

Q. What checks will be done on me and my baby?

A. Your midwife will be keeping a close eye on you and your baby for a few hours after birth, ensuring that your uterus continues to remain contracted, blood loss is normal and observations on the two of you are normal. If stitches are required, in most cases the midwife will do this in the birth room under local anaesthetic but if a tear is more extensive then an obstetrician would be required to do this in theatre under a spinal anaesthetic. She will support you to feed your baby, help you up to the shower if you can mobilise (otherwise she will help you to have a wash) and ensure you are both well before being transferred to the ward. She will also weigh your baby, offer a dose of Vitamin K and do an initial examination of the baby. A more detailed examination of your baby (NIPE exam) will take place when they are at least 6 hours old and this is performed by a midwife with additional training in this particular examination or a paediatrician. The examination includes listening for heart murmurs, checking your baby's red eye reflex, and checking for any hip dislocations. An appointment for a hearing screening will be made to ensure your baby has no problems with hearing. Further screening in the postnatal period includes the blood spot test at 5 days old where a huge list of medical conditions are screened for. These include conditions like Cystic Fibrosis, Sickle Cell and Thalassaemia and Phenylketonuria (PKU).

If your birth was straight forward, no issues have arisen immediately after birth and you feel confident with feeding your baby you can go home from the birth centre or delivery suite. In most cases though, if this is your first baby, an overnight stay may be beneficial to ensure you have support on hand with feeding your baby. If your baby was born at home the midwives will stay for a few hours after birth, ensure all is well and then leave and return either later that day or the following day. If you had a caesarean section you will most likely be in hospital for a minimum of 48 hours. The midwives are going to ensure that you can mobilise, go to the toilet without any issues, check that your wound is healing normally and that your pain relief is under control.

A postnatal check on you and the baby will be performed daily in the hospital and at each visit by the midwife once you are home. You should expect to see the midwife the day after you come out of hospital, around day five and then discharged if all is well at around day ten. At each visit the midwife will be asking you questions about feeding, how your breasts are feeling (even if you are formula feeding) to ensure you are not experiencing any difficulties and she will ask to palpate your abdomen to check your uterus is continuing to contract. She will offer to check your caesarean wound or perineal stitches to ensure everything is continuing to heal well. She will also ask if you are passing urine and opening your bowels normally. Your midwife will check your legs and look for signs of Deep Vein Thrombosis (a blood clot). Symptoms of this would be redness, one calf looking bigger than the other and tenderness. Lastly, she will remind you of the importance of postnatal pelvic floor exercises and talk to you about emotional wellbeing.

Your baby will be given a full head to toe check with your consent at each visit to ensure that there are no problems arising. She will look at your baby's skin to check for signs of jaundice or rashes. She will ask about how many dirty and wet nappies you are getting and the colour of the poo. This can be a good indicator as to how well breast feeding is going. She will also look at the baby's umbilical cord to ensure there are no signs of infection. On day five and ten the baby will be reweighed. Babies can have lost 7-8% of their birth weight on day five (more than this and a feeding assessment is required). Ideally this will be back to birth weight or not far off by day ten. If all is well your midwife will discharge you to the health visitor at around day ten. The health visitor and GP will then take over your care, although you can still contact a midwife for up to 6 weeks after birth.

Q. What are your tips for recovering from a caesarean section?

A. Recovery can be slow and challenging after a caesarean. I think people often see it as the easy way out. Trust me, it isn't. Mobilising after birth can be particularly challenging for the first week or so, and you do have to try and get up and out of bed because otherwise your body starts to seize up and then moving becomes even more painful. My advice is to take all the painkillers that are offered to you for the first week. It will help you to move about and stop severe pain when pain killers have completely worn off.

My top tips for recovery after a caesarean

-If you are breast feeding, try the rugby ball position to hold the baby. It will stop them lying across your wound. Also, have the baby and your arm supported with cushions so you are not leaning over to one side and trying to hold yourself up.

- Try and lie back and let the wound air a few times a day. You will have a little 'overhang' from where the uterus is still palpable and from swelling. By airing it you will minimise the chance of an infection.

- Use a hairdryer to dry the area after a wash. You must ensure the area stays clean and dry.

- Stitches are mostly dissolvable. Dependent on the practitioner and your body alternative options may be a 'bead stitch' which gets removed by the midwife, or staples which again the midwife usually removes at around day seven.

- Don't rush into doing any abdominal exercises until you have been given the all-clear by the GP.

- Take time to properly heal. This is major surgery and you need to give yourself plenty of time to rest and recover. We wouldn't dream about heading out to the supermarket a few days after an operation.

- If your partner needs to return to work, make sure you have help at home with you, particularly in the first few weeks.

-It will be 6 weeks until you are back driving again (or until you can apply an emergency brake). You must not lift anything heavier than the baby for 6 weeks and not be pushing the pushchair uphill.

I asked one of my clients for some more top tips on recovery and she had some other fantastic ideas I wanted to share:

1. Get support! You will need someone to bring you food and drinks and pass you things. It is really important to take time and not to rush the process.

2. Buy a litter grabber so you can pick up things out of reach!

3. Wear slip on footwear- tying laces and putting on socks is near impossible.

4. Find lots of pillows to make a nest around you so you're well supported.

5. Roll up a towel or buy a small pillow to hold against your tummy for support when you cough or sneeze.

6. Ensure you wear leggings, floaty dresses and high waisted loose clothing like gym wear- jeans are a no go as these press on the wound.

7. Frida Mom c-section pants and liners. These are high cut, disposable and great for the first two weeks (Note: normal underwear sits right on the scar line).

8. John Lewis c-section compression pants thereafter. These help you feel held in.

9. Ensure you have a changing mat upstairs and downstairs and that it is at the right height, saving you from bending down.

10. Having baby in a crib that attaches to your bed is ideal so they're within easy reach.

11. When getting out of bed swing your legs around and have something to pull yourself up with like a bed rail.

Lou's Top Tips for Self-Care:

- Delegate, delegate, delegate - don't be shy to ask your support network for help with food shopping, cooking, sibling childcare, domestic chores and laundry etc. You'll be surprised at how willing people can be to help!
- Enlist a gatekeeper - someone who can either politely turn visitors away if you're not up to visits or arrange them at a time to best suit you.
- Hydrate - ensure you drink plenty of water to help with constipation. Remember if you're breastfeeding it's thirsty work!
- If possible, sleep when baby sleeps - you are on a 24 hour shift so grab sleep whenever you can, or at the very least try to put your feet up and rest.
- Don't worry about getting dressed if you don't feel like it - stay in your pjs or **loose-fitting** clothing if it suits you. Comfort is key!
- Try a short walk - some fresh air and daylight can really lift the spirits.
- Monitor bleeding - 'Lochia' is the blood you produce after childbirth and when we are overdoing it we may notice an increased amount...your body is signalling you need to slow down.
- Have contact details of helplines/support groups/GP/Doula/Midwife close to hand for use should you need them.

> - Eat nutritious meals and snacks to replenish energy reserves and fuel your body.
> - Be kind to yourself - having a baby is a remarkable life event...it's ok if you're feeling emotional/overwhelmed/exhausted. Seek help from family, friends or a health professional if things get too much.

Tips for other caregivers

- Wash your hands before touching the baby! Babies have very immature immune systems.
- Clue up on baby sleep/hunger signals.
- Change baby's nappy.
- Offer to accompany the birthing person to appointments/support groups.
- Ensure parents are fed and watered.
- Offer to take baby for a walk so parents can rest.
- Seek help from a professional if you are concerned about anything.
- Babywear.
- Sing to baby.
- Run the hoover round/take the bin out/make parents a meal or snack.
- Take pictures of the baby and new parents. Take a breather yourself too- caring is hard work!

Preparing your other children for baby's arrival

You may be feeling a real mixture of emotions when you're expecting again and one anxiety may be over how other children in the family will react. It is inevitable that there will be bumps in the road but with some gentle preparation you can make things a little bit easier. I suggest the following to clients:

- Borrow a book about the arrival of a new baby from the library and read this with your child to introduce the idea.
- Encourage your child to help you choose some clothes and toys for the new baby so they feel involved.
- Allow your child to touch and talk to your bump if they want to.
- Talk to your child about what life will be like when the baby is here, perhaps showing them photos of them when they were a baby and what adventures they got up to!
- It is ok to be honest about babies crying and pooing. This is the reality after all!
- It is common for siblings to regress when a new member of the family comes along. Although tough, this is normal. Reassurance will need to be given to your child as they adjust.
- Buy a present for them from the baby. My daughter left a digger next to her Moses basket for her big brother!!

- Role play with dollies- explaining how gentle you need to be with them and what life is like for them in the womb.
- Don't force children to play with the new addition if they don't seem interested.
- Try to stick to your child's routine as much as possible. It can be tempting to pack siblings off to well-meaning friends and relatives, but your child will need you right now. Doing this occasionally is, of course, fine if it helps you keep your sanity but spending time with him where possible can really help, for example reading his bedtime story, doing a jigsaw together or bathing him.
- Don't introduce anything new into their world for a few months either side of your due date, such as starting nursery or potty training. This is likely to backfire otherwise.
- It is personal preference when you tell your child the news that you're expecting. Just remember that young children have no concept of time. Follow their lead; if they seem interested then answer any questions they have but otherwise don't push it.

Postnatal Plan

We are often asked to write a Birth Plan, but have you ever considered a Postnatal Plan? Surely, this stage is just as important as birth, so why don't we tend to plan for it? It can be really helpful to write down and consider some preferences so that you can share these with those within your support network, ensuring you receive the best support possible for your individual needs and wishes.

R & R

What support do I have in place to allow me to recuperate?

How easy do I find it to ask for help? What things remind me that this is important?

What do I enjoy doing that allows me to rest and take care of myself?

Nourish

My dietary requirements:

Simple, nutritious meals and snacks I enjoy:

Breakfast:

Lunch:

Dinner:

Snacks:

Drinks:

<u>Me</u>

Things that worry or concern me:

Things that are important to me and make me feel happy, confident and secure:

Our Parental Preferences

Feeding:

Sleeping:

Routine:

Nappies:

Slings/Carriers:

Contacts

Midwife:

Hospital:

GP:

Doula:

Feeding Support:

Mental health support:

Osteopath:

Support groups e.g., NCT/Facebook groups:

Chapter 15

Postnatal Doulas

What is a Postnatal Doula?

Postnatal Doulas are passionate individuals who feel extremely privileged to support families as they begin to navigate parenthood. They are empathetic, caring and patient with a keen interest in baby development and the benefits of bonding and attachment. Doulas never give advice but are there to help you make sense of everything and tune into your intuition. They offer a holistic support network, whether that is to sit chatting over a cuppa debriefing your birth experience, researching ideas with you, or enjoying baby cuddles whilst you take a shower or a long-awaited nap. Doulas provide a circle around each family offering reassurance, the latest evidence-based practise, advocating for your choices and ensuring you feel confident in your ability to parent.

Why use a Doula?

The journey into parenthood is a wonderful one but not without its challenges. New parents can be met with a barrage of advice, often conflicting, from well-meaning relatives and friends, whilst the mass of information available online can be overwhelming. A Postnatal Doula can help you decipher which information to trust at a time when you may find this difficult, especially thanks to sleep deprivation and hormones.

Adjusting to life with a newborn and the role of the parent can be daunting for many and that's where the non-judgemental support of a Doula can be invaluable. Doulas want you to feel confident in your ability to parent and are there to validate your feelings, offer you a shoulder to cry on and a listening ear.

Many new parents don't have family living close by to rely on, and the absence of a support network can feel isolating, particularly when recovering from birth and adjusting to life with a newborn. For many the practical support of a Doula can be a great solution. They can take the pressure off by providing an extra pair of hands-especially useful when partners have work commitments to juggle and/or there are other children in the family home to care for. A Doula will muck-in and adapt to put you first as you navigate your journey into parenthood in a positive way.

Choosing a Doula

When choosing a Postnatal Doula, you might find it useful to have a think first about what you're really looking for. Would you like someone to help practically- taking baby whilst you nap or shower, helping with domestic duties and preparing light meals? Are you looking for someone to support you emotionally, assisting you to find evidence-based information to help you navigate these early days? How often do you think you'll want the support of this individual? Are you keen for them to provide overnight care?

When researching Doulas it's a good idea to meet with a few to ensure you find the right fit. This is someone who is going to be involved in a very intimate and important part of your life. Choose someone who you feel you can be yourself with, who you don't mind seeing whilst in your pjs and who you feel a real connection with. Someone you believe you can talk to and who will listen unconditionally and without judgement. Perhaps start with a phone call and if all goes well suggest meeting.

It's advisable to understand whether the Doula is certified. Have they undertaken a Doula UK approved course?

A 'mentored' Postnatal Doula is worth consideration-they have been through an accredited Doula preparation course and are working towards recognition with the help of a mentor. This involves attending a certain number of postnatal jobs and feeding back on these to an experienced mentor, with the focus on progression and reflection, which can only be a good thing. Mentored Doulas are more affordable and because they have just finished their training are very keen to use what they've learnt to support new parents.

Here is a list of things a Doula can support you with. It can be really helpful to have a look through and tick which ones you feel you might need the most support with. Every family is unique and has different priorities.

☐ Preparing light meals and snacks.

☐ Light housework e.g. hoovering, laundry, washing up, ironing.

☐ Guidance on baby care.

☐ Caring for your baby, allowing you time to rest or complete other tasks.

☐ Feeding support.

☐ Signposting to the latest evidence-based information.

☐ Popping to the shops for you.

☐ Attending appointments with you.

☐ Emotional support.

☐ Babywearing.

Chapter 16

Further Reading

Books

The Social Baby- Understanding Babies' Communication from Birth- Lynne Murray

You've Got It In You: A Positive Guide to Breastfeeding- Emma Pickett

The Gentle Sleep Book- Sarah Ockwell-Smith

Sweet Sleep- La Leche League

Let's Talk About Your New Family's Sleep- Lyndsey Hookway

The Positive Breastfeeding Book- Dr Amy Brown

BabyCalm: A Guide for Happier Babies and Happier Parents- Sarah Ockwell-Smith

What Every Parent Needs to Know- Margot Sunderland

Why Mothering Matters- Maddie McMahon

Why Formula Feeding Matters- Shel Banks

Mixed up: Combination Feeding by Choice or Necessity- Lucy Ruddle

What Mothers Do- Naomi Stadlen

Websites

National Childbirth Trust www.nct.org.uk 0300 330 0700

BASIS Baby Sleep Information Source www.basisonline.org.uk

Lullaby Trust www.lullabytrust.org.uk

Lactation Consultants of Great Britain www.lcgb.org.uk

Association of Breastfeeding Mothers www.amb.me.uk 0300 3305453

La Leche League www.laleche.org.uk 0345 120 2918

BreastfeedingNetwork
www.breastfeedingnetwork.org.uk 0300 1000212

Breastfeeding.support https://breastfeeding.support

United Kingdom Association of Milk Banking www.ukamb.org

Association of Tongue Tie Practitioners www.tongue-tie.org.uk

UNICEF   www.unicef.org

World Health Organisation https://www.who.int

NHS www.nhs.uk

Stillbirth and Neonatal Death Society www.sands.org.uk
0808 164 3332

Cry-sis www.cry-sis.org.uk

Pre and Postnatal Depression Advice and Support
www.pandasfoundation.org.uk 0808 1961 776

Birth Trauma Association
www.birthtraumaassociation.org.uk

The Multiple Births Association
https://www.multiplebirths.org.uk/

Twins Trust www.twinstrust.org

Doula UK www.doula.org.uk

Netmums Parenting Community www.netmums.co.uk

Carrying Matters, Rosie Knowles
www.carryingmatters.co.uk

UK Sling Libraries www.ukslinglibraries.wordpress.com

Brazelton www.brazelton.co.uk

Lou Hirst www.doula-lou.com

Hannah Croft IBCLC www.hannahcroft-ibclc.co.uk

Kathryn Stagg IBCLC www.kathrynstaggibclc.com

Hannah Ewin, Birth Boutique www.birthboutique.co.uk

First Steps Nutrition www.firststepsnutrition.org

Instagram

@doulalouuk
@hannahcroftibclc
@olivia_lactation_consultant
@kathrynstaggibclc
@osteokarly
@carolsmyth_ibclc_cbt
@basis_babysleepinfosource
@theslingconsultancy
@carryingmatters
@lullabytrust
@sarahockwellsmith
@lyndsey_hookway
@birthboutique

Apps

Global Health Media, Birth & Beyond
BASIS Infant Sleep

Ingram Content Group UK Ltd.
Milton Keynes UK
UKHW020814060623
422954UK00016B/1036